God Wants You Healthy!

How the Genesis Diet
Gives You Health, Healing
and Longevity

by
Dennis Urbans, BASc

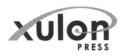

xulon
PRESS

God Wants You Healthy!
by Dennis Urbans, BASc

For Worldwide Distribution
Printed in the United States of America

Library of Congress Cataloging-in-Publication Data —
Urbans, Dennis, 1959 -
Includes Index.
ISBN 1-59781-463-6

www.xulonpress.com

DEDICATION

Dedicated to my wife Heather and children Katrina, Daniel and Joshua for their support, understanding and joining with me to become Genesis 1:29 vegetarians.

FOREWORD

Most Western countries today are reporting that the number one health problem in their respective populations is obesity. If that is not the greatest health challenge to us then it will be other recurrent diseases related to what we eat. Research shows that immigrants from other societies which are historically unaffected by traditional recurrent western health problems, become so in a relatively short time as they indulge in the western diet.

Major international food outlets already smarting under the glare of litigation are changing what they sell to provide choice and avoid future court cases.

Clearly what we eat and how we exercise is directly related to physical health outcomes. A huge commercial industry has emerged to assist with dieting and exercise. Special foods may be home delivered to help the busy urbanite eat better with even less time to prepare nutritious foods now that regular visits to the local gymnasium have to be squeezed into already overcrowded schedules. If there is any spare time then there are DVD's to watch, CD's to listen to and many, many books to read regarding healthier eating habits. So why another one?

Dennis Urbans had a very serious personal health crisis. That set him on a personal search over some years to see if his problems could be solved through basic life style changes, especially food intake, instead of persevering with standard medical responses. What he discovered and has practiced in his family now for a number of years, has revolutionized his health and life. This book is the result of his search and personal successful experimentation.

Following Dennis' recommendations could be the cheapest way out of your health challenges. It may also improve the quality of your life as well as extending it. Being fit on earth might also just fit you out for Heaven — if you follow the manufacturer's manual — the Bible.

Dr Stuart Robinson
Senior Pastor
Crossway Baptist Church, Melbourne, Australia
www.crossway.org.au

God Wants You Healthy! describes a solution to the most critical nutrition-related diseases we face—a low-fat plant-based diet. Mr. Urbans not only justifies why a vegan diet is crucial for health but also gives helpful hints and practical advice for adopting this kind of nutritious regimen.

Jennifer K. Reilly, R.D.
Managing Director
The Cancer Project, Washington D.C.
www.cancerproject.org

ABOUT THE AUTHOR

In October 2000, at the age of 41, I presented into hospital with diabetes. My sugar levels were 25+ (some 5 times the normal level). I was obese and had a number of health issues such as constant reflux, blurring vision, high blood pressure, tiredness, and all the other complications that come with the disease.

From this shock, I decided to study health and nutrition from a Biblical point of view, as well as from secular material. As a keen supporter of Biblical Creationism, Genesis 1:29 jumped out at me as a key verse...

And God said, See, I have given you every herb that yields seed which is on the face of the earth, and every tree whose fruit yields seed; to you it shall be for food. And it was so. Genesis 1:29

And it all seemed to make sense. If God originally created and instructed us to be vegetarians, why wouldn't eating such a diet be the healthiest for us? I had everything to gain and nothing to lose. If it didn't work, I would just have to live the diabetic life and try to keep it under control as best as possible. But if it did work, what a terrific testimony to the Word of God that would be!

And it did work! When animal products such as meat, dairy and eggs were removed from the table, and a diet based on the fruits, vegetables, legumes and whole grains was embraced, my blood sugar levels began to plummet back to normal levels in only a period of four months. I was also able to gradually reduce my daily insulin injections, and finally able to remove them altogether. By the time of my six monthly checkup at the hospital, I was happy to report to the doctors that I was insulin free and drug free, to their amazement. In that period, I began to lose weight, and in the 12 months after that, I lost a total of about 30 kg, and have continued to maintain a weight level around 90kg. My blood sugar levels are consistently and daily within normal levels.

In a way, becoming a diabetic was a fortuitous experience. It made me take a good look at my diet-style, and this book is a result of that experience. It is amazing how the Lord can turn your life around. Without His intervention, I would have been, for sure, a heart attack victim at an early age.

CONTENTS

PREFACE

It can be seen time and time again. Honest, hard-working men and women of God being struck down by sickness and disease, ending or curtailing the work God intended them to do. Why should these people become so sick? Did God make a mistake?

Disease not only affects the people afflicted, but families, friends and church community as well, and sometimes for very long periods of time. How can this be if God promises us health and longevity? Did God make a mistake?

Furthermore, millions of people of all ages, including children, are suffering from long term illness such as asthma, hay fever, allergies, sinusitis, back-pain, arthritis, hypertension, just to name a few. Diseases unheard of in children a generation ago, such as Type 2 diabetes, are now becoming more and more prevalent. What a dismal picture this is. Did God make a mistake?

Not only that, many people both young and old suffer daily in their lives simply because they are too tired and lethargic to reach their full potential. As a nation we are getting fatter and less healthy, with seemingly no end in sight.

There are many promises in the Bible regarding good

health and longevity of life. How can we take these promises seriously when we see so much premature death and disease around us? Wouldn't it be amazing, instead, to see God's people active and vibrant well into their 80's and more? Imagine how much work could be done for the Lord by healthy, vivacious and active seniors. What a testimony this would be to the world!

However, we humans can be strange creatures, often ignoring important warning signs until we come to a crisis in our health. Hopefully, at that point, it is not too late.

Good health is our personal responsibility. Ultimately, God charges the responsibility for our health to each of us. Looking after our body is itself a form of worship and sacrifice to Him who created us, to ultimately present ourselves blameless to Him. No, God did not make a mistake. It is us who have made the mistake!

Can we collectively rise to the challenge of better health? Will we decide to no longer be ignorant about how to look after ourselves? Will we tame our eating habits in line with God's word?

This book provides a Biblical basis to diet and lifestyle that will help sustain good health and vitality well into our senior years. I pray that you can spend a few hours of your time reading this book and consider the principles described within it. It will change your life!

And above all...

Beloved, I pray that you may prosper in all things and be in health, just as your soul prospers. 3 John 2

Chapter 1
MARVELOUS ARE HIS WORKS

The book of Genesis is the foundational book of the Bible. In this marvelous record, we find a true and reliable account of the origin of all things: the universe, the solar system, the earth, mankind and even the origin of evil and sin. If the Bible is true, then its foundation must also be true.

Perfection of Creation

During the creation week, by the power of His word, God created all things to perfection. This is affirmed by the words "it was good" being repeated at the end of each Creation day, and then the term "it was very good" at the end of the sixth day, before God rested.

Then God saw everything that He had made, and indeed it was very good. Genesis 1:31

Everything was perfect and everything was in its place. The earth was created a fully functional biosphere, supporting an abundance of life from the smallest microbes to the greatest sea creatures and giant land animals, as well as man himself.

Having just formed Adam from the chemical elements

found in the earth, God "breathed into his nostrils the breath of life" (Genesis 2:7) in order to activate his bodily functions.

God, who made the world and everything in it, since He is Lord of heaven and earth, does not dwell in temples made with hands. Nor is He worshipped with men's hands, as though He needed anything, since He gives to all life, breath, and all things. Acts 17:24-25

In the midst of all this marvelous creation, God himself planted and prepared a special place where Adam and his wife Eve would dwell and live forever in a sinless state — the Garden of Eden. Here, every tree "pleasant to the sight and good for food" was planted for man's benefit.

God also explained the reason for being created: simply to be fruitful and multiply, to fill the earth and subdue it (Genesis 1:28). He is the giver of life, and it can come from no other source. He is the original source of life, He is the sustainer of life, and He sent Jesus to die for our sins so that we "may have life, and have it more abundantly" (John 10:10).

From the Earth

Of the one hundred plus elements listed in the Periodic Table, ninety are naturally occurring in the "dust of the ground," and more than one quarter of these are found in our bodies. Some elements, such as cobalt, iodine, magnesium, iron and chromium occur in very small amounts, but have significant and complex roles.

The first man was of the earth, made of dust. The second Man is the Lord from Heaven. 1 Corinthians 15:47

The more abundant elements exist as chemical compounds, the most notable being water (H_2O) making up some 70% of our bodies.[1] Carbon, hydrogen and oxygen atoms combine in different ways to form carbohydrates such as sugars, fats and glycogen. Carbon, hydrogen, oxygen, nitrogen and phosphorous form more complex molecules such as amino acids, proteins and the amazingly complex DNA structures that ultimately determine our unique physical characteristics.[2]

Fearfully and Wonderfully Made

Every organ, every chemical, biological and physical process, every mental, emotional and spiritual faculty are all designed to work in harmony for each of us to live, work, love, play and praise Him who created us.

> **For You formed my inner parts. You covered me in my mother's womb. I will praise You, for I am fearfully and wonderfully made. Marvelous are Your works, and that my soul knows very well. My frame was not hidden from You when I was made in secret and skillfully wrought in the lowest parts of the earth. Your eyes saw my substance, being yet unformed. And in your book they all were written. The days fashioned for me when as yet there were none of them. Psalm 139:13-16**

At the physical, chemical and biological level, our human body created by God is an amazing self-replicating and self-repairing machine, a marvel of biological engineering.

> **He has made everything beautiful in its time. Also He has put eternity in their hearts, except that no one can find out the work that God does from beginning to end. Ecclesiastes 3:11**

Ernst Haeckel, a German physician in the 19th century, abandoned his practice in 1859 after reading Charles

Darwin's book Origin of Species. He is infamous for his now debunked "law of capitulation" where growing embryos supposedly pass through various stages of evolution. Haeckal believed that a cell was a "simple little lump of albuminous combination of carbon."[3]

But the cell is far from basic. It is a marvelous and complex structure in its own right. Scientists have been examining cells for many years and yet we still do not fully comprehend all its amazing complexities. Some 10 to 100 trillion cells make up each and every component of our bodies.[4]

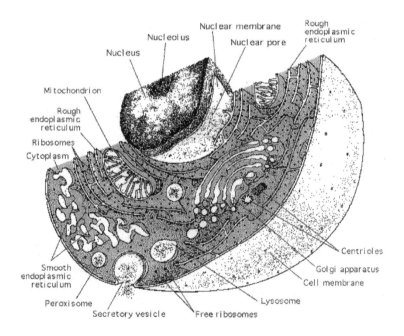

The cell is certainly not basic. It consists of 30,000 genes per chromosome, with 22 chromosomes plus X and Y sex-determining chromosomes. Some chromosomes contain up to 300 million nucleic acid "bases," with each base joined to its neighbor in precise order. Each gene interacts with four or five others, on average. Diagram courtesy of the National Human Genome Research Institute.

Since the discovery of the double helix DNA molecule fifty years ago, genome science has advanced rapidly. The Human Genone Project, completed in April 2003, was a huge international research effort to map the genes of the human cell, giving us the blueprint for the building of the human body.[5] All this research has verified the extreme complexity of the cell, a far cry from Haeckel's lump of albuminous[6] combination of carbon! This could only come from intelligent design and an intelligent Designer.

Cells form many complex and specific components in the body. These components work intricately together to form hundreds of systems all interacting together in amazing and perfect synergy. To assert that hundreds of individual bodily systems, all working together in perfect unison and harmony, came about by chance random mutation is fantasy and falsehood of the highest order. It is for these reasons that we reject evolution and embrace the marvelous record of Creation found in the book of Genesis.

> **O Timothy! Guard what was committed to your trust, avoiding the profane and idle babblings and contradictions of what is falsely called knowledge. By professing it some have become strayed concerning the faith. 1 Timothy 6:20-21**

Even today, many of these systems are not well understood by medical and anatomical scientists.

Skeletal System

The skeletal system protects organs such as the brain, lungs and heart, gives the body shape, enables movement as muscles contract, and provides the manufacture of blood cells in the marrow.

In an adult there are 206 separate bones, connected to each other by ligaments at the joints. Bone tissue is very much a living component of the body, having its own nerves and blood vessels. Some 2.6 million blood cells are produced every second to replace spent cells destroyed by the liver.[7]

Bones are also like a bank for some minerals, particularly calcium and phosphorous. When an excess of these minerals exists in the blood, they are stored in the bones, but when these mineral levels are low, they will be withdrawn to replenish supply.[8]

Muscular System

Muscles are special tissues that contract when signals supplied by the brain are transmitted via the nervous system. Since the muscles are attached to bones, the contraction results in bodily movement. Because muscles can only pull, not push, most are arranged in opposing pairs.

There are 650 separate muscles in the body.[9] Voluntary muscles enable movement of the limbs as a result of our thoughts from the brain, while involuntary muscles, such as the heart, diaphragm and intestines are automatically controlled, even when asleep.

Respiratory System

Oxygen enters the respiratory system through the mouth and nose, passing through the trachea into the lungs via bronchial tubes. Some 600 million tiny sacs called alveoli are surrounded by capillaries where oxygen is transferred to the blood and carbon dioxide is extracted from the blood.[10]

The diaphragm is the main muscle that controls breathing. As the diaphragm flattens, it creates a vacuum in the lungs which draws in air through the mouth or nose to the lungs via the trachea. When it collapses, the chest compresses, forcing out the spent air containing carbon dioxide.[11]

Circulatory System

The average adult has about 5 liters of blood flowing through many kilometers of veins, arteries and capillaries.[12] Oxygen breathed into the lungs is exchanged for spent gases (mainly carbon dioxide) in the air sacs in the lungs and capillary vessels surrounding them.

Little is wasted in the economy of the blood. The 5 million red blood cells destroyed every second are broken down into their base materials for re-use in the construction of new cells.

White blood cells, or leucocytes, are the body's fighting force against the attacks of bacteria and other foreign matter.[13] When a foreign invader enters the body, the white blood cells mobilize and counterattack. For open sores and infection, bone marrow produces additional white blood cells to cope with the emergency.

Lymphatic System

Lymph is a transparent fluid containing white blood cells and forms part of the autoimmune defense system. Unlike blood that is pumped by the heart, lymph fluid relies on muscular movement to move itself around the body. It is therefore important to exercise regularly in order to ensure efficient circulation and functionality of the lymphatic system.[14]

Along the lymph network are lymph nodes that serve as filters for harmful substances, as well as producing immune cells to fight disease. A number of organs, such as the tonsils, adenoids, spleen and thymus form part of the lymph system.

Nervous System

The nervous system is a complex network of transmitters that send and receive messages to and from the brain. The spinal cord contains a thick set of nerves branching out to all parts of the body.

The nervous system is divided into two parts: the Somatic Nervous System which controls motor axons that signal muscular movement, and the Autonomic Nervous System that regulates organ functions that are not subject to voluntary control, such as the heart and intestines.[15]

The brain, of course, is the center of the nervous system and all that occurs within the body, and is more powerful than any computer ever built. It contains an estimated 100 billion neurons (brain cells), with each neuron averaging some 10,000 connections each. There exists an amazing network totaling 90 million meters of neural fibers.[16] Even today, how thoughts and desires originate is still not well understood.

Digestive System

Food provides fuel to live, energy to work and play, and raw materials to build new cells. Food is mechanically and chemically broken down by the digestive system and transported to every part of the body by the blood via the circulatory system.

The stomach lining and pancreas produce strong digestive juices (principally hydrochloric acid, gastric juices and mucus) that chemically react with food, breaking it down into its constituent components. The gall bladder produces bile to assist the digestion of fats.[17]

Some 6 meters of small intestine continue to chemically break down food, now converted by the stomach into chyme, allowing nutrients to pass through the intestinal walls and be picked up by the blood. From here, nutrients such as carbohydrates, lipids and amino acids are transported to the liver to be processed, stored and distributed as required.

Any remaining useful substances are absorbed through the walls of the large intestines. It is also in the large intestine where spent debris and dead cells are absorbed into the bulk, which is formed into feces ready for evacuation.

Reproductive System

Testes located in the scrotum produce sperm. Since normal body temperature is lethal to sperm, the scrotum is located outside the body where the temperature is some 3° Celsius cooler.[18]

When the male ejaculates, the sperm travels from the scrotum then behind the bladder into the urethra and finally exiting the penis into the female vagina. In the female, there are some 300,000 precursor eggs called follicles. Of these, only about 300 will ever be released as ovum for fertilization in the fallopian tube by the male sperm.[19]

The fertilized ovum, now called the zygote, attaches itself to the wall of the uterus and begins the process of fetal development. After about 40 weeks, the baby will be ready for birth through the vagina.

Human Longevity

Human longevity has long been a puzzle and fascination. Today, there is much scientific endeavor devoted to living longer, as well as life extension societies and even magazines. Ponce de Leon, a Spanish explorer who sailed with Christopher Columbus, searched for the so-called Fountain of Youth after hearing stories about certain springs that supposedly kept people young (this Fountain of Youth has never been found).

However, God said that man would not live longer than 120 years, and even today with modern scientific and medical knowledge, this is the practical maximum that a human can live. The oldest authenticated age at death is 122 years 164 days for a woman and 120 years 237 days for a man.[20]

And the Lord said, My spirit shall not strive with man forever, for he is indeed flesh; yet his days shall be one hundred and twenty years. Genesis 6:3

When Adam and Eve sinned against God, not only did man become separated from God, but no longer was the tree of life available to sustain immortality. Death surely did come, for God said, "For dust you are, and to dust you shall return" (Genesis 3:19). Even, so humans in Adam's time lived an average of some 900 years.

Immediately after the Flood, however, a dramatic decrease in human longevity occurred. Noah managed 950 years, but his son, Shem, only 600. The following graph shows rapidly decreasing longevity after the Great Flood in Noah's day…

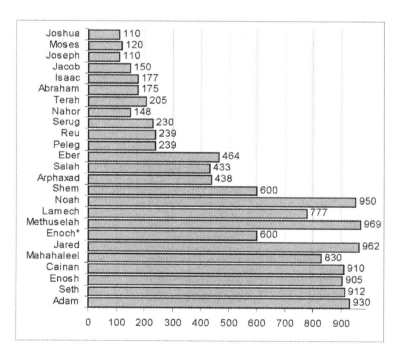

* Enoch did not die, but was translated directly to heaven.

A number of factors can be attributed to this decline in longevity. Prior to the Flood, there was no rain (Genesis 2:5) and the atmosphere was both uniformly stable and warm. Harmful solar energy outside the visible spectrum, such as ultra-violet, infrared, gamma and x-ray radiation where efficiently filtered out by the expanse of water above the atmosphere that God called sky (Genesis 1:7-8). After the Flood, this protective water layer no longer existed, allowing this harmful electromagnetic radiation to penetrate to the earth's surface.

The lush vegetation that God created, albeit now infested with thorns and thistles, was totally wiped out by the Flood resulting in huge reserves of crude oil, natural gas and coal we exploit today. Such lush vegetation provided the service of oxygenating the atmosphere to a much higher level than is possible today. Oxygen, the "breathe of life" (Genesis 2:7), is required by the body to react with the products of digestion to provide muscles and tissues with energy.

One of the effects of the rapid upheavals of the earth at the time of the Flood, as well as the continuous erosion effects of moving water, was the leaching out of vital minerals and trace elements required for sustaining long and healthy life. Concentrations of these minerals and trace elements in soils and plants grown today are lower than that which existed before the Flood.

The consumption of animal flesh was only now authorized by God (Genesis 9:3) no doubt as a provision for Noah and his family to obtain sustenance until the earth was again filled with vegetation. However, the eating of animal flesh became all too common, requiring God to pronounce a number of dietary restrictions for the sake of the health of His people (refer the book of Leviticus) and to ensure that the life of the flesh — the blood — was not to be consumed, but retained for sacrifice and atonement for the soul (Leviticus 17:11).

Despite the maximum age capped at 120 years, the average age at death in the Western world is about 77.6 years (this number varies from country to country).[21] Moreover, the shocking statistic is that the majority of men and woman die of heart attacks, strokes, cancers, diabetes, and organ diseases. Few people die of a natural ripe old age. Why is this so?

The following table shows the number of deaths by disease in the United States in the year 2002...[22]

Disease	No. Deaths	Percent
Heart disease	696,947	28.5%
Malignant neoplasms (cancer)	557,271	22.8%
Cerebrovascular disease (stroke)	162,672	6.6%
Chronic lower respiratory diseases	124,816	5.2%
Accidents	106,802	4.4%
Diabetes mellitus	73,249	3.0%
Influenza and pneumonia	65,681	2.7%
Alzheimers disease	58,866	2.4%

God does not desire that any of His people live and die in agony, but rather, we should live a full life to the end of our days. Many Scriptures affirm this...

You shall walk in the ways which the Lord your God has commanded you, that you may live and that it may be well with you, and that you may prolong your days, in the land which you shall possess. Deuteronomy 5:33

That your days and the days of your children may be multiplied in the land of which the Lord swore to your fathers to give them, like the days of the heavens above the earth. Deuteronomy 11:21

So if you walk in My ways, to keep My statutes and My commandments, as your father David walked, then I will lengthen your days. 1 Kings 3:14

You shall come to the grave at a full age, as a shear of grain ripens in its seasons. Job 5:26

I have come that they may have life, and that they might have it more abundantly. John 10:10

Consider Moses, whose eyes were not weak, nor was his strength diminished at his death at 120 years (Deuteronomy 34:7) and King David, who died full of age and riches and honor (1 Chronicles 29:28). Even today, there are some people groups who characteristically live between 100 and 120 years in excellent health.

Can you imagine living in a land where nobody gets cancer, heart disease, ulcers or appendicitis? Can you imagine a group of people where everybody has perfect 20/20 vision, even in old age? Such a group is the Hunzakuts of Northern Pakistan, as reported by Dr Alexander Leaf on assignment with National Geographic...[23]

The energy and endurance of the Hunzakuts can probably be credited as much to what they don't eat as what they do eat. First of all, they don't eat a great deal of anything. The United States Department of Agriculture estimates that the average daily food intake for Americans of all ages amounts to 3,300 calories, with 100 grams of protein, 157 grams of fat and 380 grams of carbohydrates. In contrast, studies by Pakistani doctors show that adult males of Hunza consume a little more than 1,900 calories daily, with only 50 grams of protein, 36 grams of fat, and 354 grams of carbohydrates. Both the protein and fat are largely of vegetable origin. [Dr Alexander Leaf]

Dr Allen Banik, optometrist and author of Hunza Land, examined the eyes of the Hunza's oldest citizens and found them to have excellent eyesight.[24]

Human longevity is a complex issue, and many factors are involved. Even belonging to a vibrant church can increase your life! A study of 4,000 elderly North Carolina residents by Duke University found that those who attended religious services weekly had a 25% lower death rate.[25] Religious attendance also works through increased social ties and behavioral factors to decrease the risks of death. And although the magnitude of the association between religious attendance and mortality varies by cause of death, the association is consistent across causes.[26]

However, Christians should not rest on these laurels. Although attending church and shunning behavioral factors such as smoking and drinking alcohol most certainly helps with health and longevity, there is still a propensity for western Christians to eat diets high in fats, oils, sugar and salt. In the next chapter, we will examine the Genesis Diet and its effect on health and well-being.

Chapter 2
THE GENESIS DIET

Having just created Adam and Eve, and explaining to them their purpose and responsibility on the earth, God clearly told them what they were to eat: unprocessed, raw fruits and vegetables, nuts, seeds and grains. The Genesis Diet is therefore a pure vegetarian diet, and relates most closely to today's vegan diet (in particular, a raw food vegetarian diet).

> **And God said, See, I have given you every herb that yields seed which is on the face of the earth, and every tree whose fruit yields seed; to you it shall be for food. And it was so. Genesis 1:29**

This same nutritional regimen was also to be shared by God's creatures as well. There can be no doubt — both man and animals were created vegetarian, with all sustenance coming purely from plant sources.

> **Also, to every beast of the earth, to every bird of the air, and to everything that creeps on the earth, in which there is life, I have given every green herb for food, and it was so. Genesis 1:30**

Why did God specifically give mankind and animals this nutritional regimen? If nutrition is not important, why then did God mention it at all? The answer, of course, is that God gives us instructions and commandments that are for our own good. How far we have removed ourselves from His original design and purpose!

The entire western diet is unbalanced and lacks sufficient vitamins and minerals for good health. If there is any axiom in nutrition, it is that a diet rich in fruits and vegetables reduces the risk of heart diseases, cancers, diabetes and other chronic diseases. The following table shows how the typical western diet differs enormously from the ideal proportions obtainable from the Genesis Diet (in percentage by calories)…

Component	Western Diet	Ideal Proportion
Fat	30 to 50%	10%
Carbohydrates	20 to 35%	80%
Protein	25 to 30%	10%
Fiber	10 to 20 grams	50 to 60 grams
Vitamins	Deficient	Sufficient
Minerals	Deficient	Sufficient
Cholesterol	500 mg per day	Zero

Of course, the best defense against diseases such as cancer, heart disease, stroke and diabetes is not to get them in the first place. The Genesis Diet dramatically reduces the chance of contracting these diseases, and increases the length of human life. It contains a full arsenal of powerful plant nutrients (known as phytonutrients) that contain natural protective chemicals able to be utilized effectively by our complex defensive and regenerative mechanisms.

Our Responsibility

After a torrid start to the last century, with World War I, the Great Depression and World War II, the 1950's saw a surge in optimism, scientific endeavor, inventions, and economic and social restructuring. Professor Harvey Levenstein, a social historian who studied the changing patterns of the American diet, describes the 1950's as The Golden Age of Food Processing, where all sorts of food processing methods made life easier for each and every housewife.[1] There were even restaurants where customers would cook their frozen meals in tableside microwave ovens. The age of fast-food was born.

As a result, fatty, junk and processed foods are now being eaten with great abundance and abandonment, without much thought or consideration to the damage they are doing. It is now considered normal to drive to our favorite fast-food restaurant, queue up for quick service, pay a few dollars, and sit down to eat a meal. When middle age comes, after 30 or 40 years of eating diets high in fats, cholesterol, sugars and salts, all manner of diseases such as heart attacks, strokes, diabetes and cancers begin to appear. Christians in their 40's, 50's, 60's and even older should be at their spiritual prime, but many are bogged down by sickness and disease they should not have!

At the household level, Scripture warns us against being idle in our food and meal preparation. How far removed are we from God's ways! Abrogating family responsibility by excessive eating at fast food restaurants is not only potentially detrimental to health, but it is not how God intended us to prepare meals.

She watches over the ways of her household, and does not eat the bread of idleness. Proverbs 31:27

Also, many spend their money on expensively packaged food, when instead we would benefit more by simply eating an apple! Despite eating and eating more, we are no more satisfied.

Why do you spend money for what is not bread, and your wages for what does not satisfy? Listen diligently to Me, and eat what is good, and let your soul delight itself in abundance. Isaiah 55:2

An honest appraisal in the church today would find many afflicted with ongoing diseases, suffering a lack of vitality and vibrancy. If Christians worship a healing God, then why isn't healthier and longer life being experienced as He intended?

God considers our physical bodies as temples (literally a dwelling place) of the Holy Spirit. After all, He "fearfully and wonderfully" created them.

Do you not know that your body is the temple of the Holy Spirit who is in you, whom you have from God? 1 Corinthians 6:19

We therefore have a responsibility to ensure that which we allow to enter our bodies, both spiritually and physically, is not harmful to us, so that we can be strong for the work of the Lord. Ailing Christians do not work well for the Lord, and require considerable resources that could be better deployed for His harvest. There are clear warnings in Scripture that we are entirely responsible for our own health.

Now therefore, thus says the Lord of hosts; Consider you ways! You have sown much, and bring in little; you eat, but do not have enough; you drink, but you are not filled with drink; you clothe yourselves, but no one is warm; and he who earns wages, earns wages

**to put into a bag with holes. Thus says the
Lord of hosts: Consider your ways! Haggai
1:6-7**

While medical science has helped man in many ways, it is no substitute, and never will be a substitute, for God's proper eating and health management.

Knowing the cause of disease means their curse can be avoided.

**Like a flitting sparrow, like a flying swallow,
so a curse without cause shall not alight.
Proverbs 26:2**

How we treat our bodies on a continuous and daily basis has a very powerful effect on our health and quality of life. A diet based on Genesis 1:29 requires few doctors' appointments, minimal agonizing periods in waiting rooms, virtually no cutting open of the body and taking bits out, minimal ingestion of (potentially harmful) medicines, and minimal jabbing with needles!

During the past five decades, there have been some 250 research studies on various aspects of Seventh-Day Adventist health showing the benefits of their vegetarian diet and life style. These studies have confirmed SDA longevity greater than the general population, eg, 8.9 years in California, 8.9 years in Holland, 4.2 years in Norway and 9.5 years in Poland.[2]

Even back in 1973, Dr Sidney Katz, Professor of Pharmacology at the University of British Columbia, recognized the generally better health of Seventh Day Adventists...[3]

*I've got some advice on how to improve the
health of Canadians and, at the same time,
lop billions of dollars off our annual health
costs. I think we should study the lifestyle of*

adherents of the Seventh-day Adventist Church and then explore ways and means of persuading the public to emulate the Adventists in at least some ways. [Dr Sidney Katz]

Better public hygiene, such as running tap water and piped sewerage, have contributed immensely to the health and well being of the population. In centuries past, when hygiene standards were nowhere near that of modern society, many outbreaks of deadly diseases occurred. One notable example is the Bubonic plaque, otherwise known as the Black Death. This deadly disease has occurred from time to time over the centuries, in particular in 1334 when an esti-mated three quarters of Europe's population died, and again in 1665 when thousands died in the great plague of London.[4]

Great advances in medicine have been made in the past century. One example is penicillin originally obtained from mould of the genus penicillium,[5] but is now made syntheti-cally. Mass immunization has all but eradicated many diseases such as diphtheria, pertussis (whooping cough), tetanus, poliomyelitis, measles and rubella, amongst many others.[6] All these are great advances that today we can sometimes take very much for granted.

But even in our modern, cleaner, medically advanced world, we still see so much obesity, illness and disease.

Health Spending

It comes as no surprise that the amount of money spent on health care has grown rapidly in the past few decades. Health expenditure as a percentage of Gross Domestic Product (GDP) has risen significantly over the past few years. The Organization of Economic Co-operation and Development (OECD) has recognized and reported this trend to higher and higher health spending...[7]

Spending on health and healthcare in most OECD countries has risen dramatically over the past five years. Combined with lower economic growth, the increase in health spending has driven the share of health expenditure as a percentage of GDP up from an average 7.8% in 1997 to 8.5% in 2002. This is in sharp contrast to the period 1992 to 1997, when the share of GDP spent on health remained almost unchanged. [OECD]

In the United States, health spending as a proportion of GDP is even higher, with 14.9% of GDP in 2002, up from 13.3% in 2000. This represents about $5,440 per person. Furthermore, annual total increases ranged from 7.1% in 2000, 8.5% in 2001 and 9.3% in 2002, reaching $1.5 trillion.[8]

How can such increasing spending on health be sustained into the future, particularly when society is ageing as rapidly as it is? Within the next 50 years, the number of people over 60 years of age will outnumber people under 15.[9]

There is much uncertainty in government about economic, health and social welfare policies directed towards the aged and ageing population. According to the US Census Bureau, the population of Americans over 65 years of age will be 53 million in 2020. As a proportion of population, this will represent and increase from 12.6% in 2000 to 16.5% in 2020.[10]

Of course, ageing is not a crime, and each and every human being is entitled to grow old with grace and dignity, having endured through life's trials and tribulations. But unfortunately, for most of us, our twilight years will become a battle against some lifestyle disease such as heart disease, stroke, cancer, respiratory problems, dementia and the like.

Does it make sense to work hard all your life, only to spend your entire savings for somebody to cut you open and implant a dead person's heart?

The problem is not really that we have an insufficient number of doctors, hospitals, clinics, money, medicines or scientific medical knowledge. Rather, the problem is that we have too many sick people, particularly the elderly. On the basis of prevailing cancer incidence rates, it is expected that the number of cancer cases will double from 1.3 million in 2000 to 2.5 million in 2050. Moreover, the number of cancer patients over 85 is expected to increase four-fold in the same period.[11]

Building more hospitals and clinics, training more doctors and surgeons, throwing more money at more research and spending more on public and private health insurance will not alleviate the problem of an increasing health burden. This is reactive health care, not preventative. Indeed, such an approach to health more likely increases health costs.

For example, fifty years ago a heart attack most assuredly meant that the victim would, unfortunately, pass away and require nothing more than a burial. Today, however, if the victim is attended to quickly enough, complex coronary bypasses, angioplasties (where catheters are inserted into arteries and inflated to open them up) and even heart transplants are normally performed. Such procedures are not without risk, and patients do not just walk out the hospital door like nothing has happened.

For a start, the risk of dying during a coronary bypass operation is five to ten percent.[12] In the case of balloon angioplasties, some 25 to 50% of all cases, blood vessels become blocked again due to restenosis, or the formation of new atherosclerotic plaques. These occur because blood-clotting agents form a thrombosis over the wounded vessel, which can become large enough to close off the artery completely.[13]

Of the patients that do not die, nearly all suffer some degree of brain damage by the heart-lung machine that keeps them alive during the operation. Between 15 and 44% experience permanent brain damage after bypass surgery. Other risks include the possibility of arterial plaques breaking loose from arterial walls and lodging themselves in arteries serving the brain, causing stroke. As for heart transplant patients (as well as lung, kidney and other transplants), medications must be taken for life in order to stop the new organ from being rejected. These medicines are very strong, making it much harder to fight off infections. They raise blood pressure (hypertension) and increase the risk of lymphoma, a form of cancer that affects the cells of the immune system.[14]

DNA Manipulation

Despite all the risks, organ transplantation is now a very common procedure even though only performed as a last resort. However, the problem is a chronic shortage of donor organs against an ever-increasing demand for them. Perversely, the success of road safety campaigns and the decline in road deaths has contributed to organ donation numbers dropping.

One solution being researched is xenotransplantation (xeno meaning stranger, or foreigner). This is the genetic modification of animals, particularly pigs, for the harvesting of their organs to be transplanted into humans. Without surprise, this research raises immense passion amongst animal rights activists, theologians, ethicists and medical professionals.

The biggest hurdle with xenotransplantation is rejection of the transplanted organ. The body's rejection mechanism is so effective that hyperacute rejection simply destroys any non-modified organ implanted in the human body. This is the greatest hurdle in making xenotransplantation a reality.[15]

This Frankenstein approach to medicine is a nightmare waiting to happen. The risk of animal diseases entering the human population is too great a risk to contemplate. How wise was God who created each creature unique...

> **So God created great sea creatures and every living thing that moves, with which the waters abounded, according to their kind, and every winged bird according to its kind. And God saw that it was good. Genesis 1:21**

Selective breeding has been with us for thousands of years. Jacob cunningly used selective breeding techniques with Laban's goats to his own benefit (Genesis 30:37-43). However, selective breeding does not cross over the boundaries of species, does not create another species of animal or plant, and certainly does not involve splicing DNA from one species into another, even between plants and animals. In some cases, cross-breeding of two similar varieties of one species can produce a slightly different variety of the same species, but never a new species. There are certainly strict limits to how far variations within a species can go. God has placed a DNA barrier between all species, a non-transmutability of kinds created by Him.

> **You shall keep My statutes. You shall not let your livestock breed with another kind. You shall not sow your field with mixed seed, nor shall a garment of mixed linen and wool come upon you. Leviticus 19:19**

Not content to work within the laws of nature given to us from God, we have now decided to develop technologies that alter the very genetic makeup of living organisms such as plants, animals and bacteria. Combining DNA from different organisms is known as recombinant DNA technology, cell fusion, and gene deletion and doubling. The resultant organism is said to be genetically modified, genetically engineered or transgenic.[16]

By 2003, some 68 million hectares of land in over 18 countries were growing genetically modified crops, mainly soybean, corn, cotton and canola. Currently being developed is a banana that contains human vaccines against infectious diseases such as hepatitis B, fruit and nut trees that yield years earlier, and plants that produce new types of plastics.[17]

The main driver of genetic modification is commercial benefit, and the main beneficiaries of such technology are the companies that produce and market genetically modified seeds and chemicals. These companies are also taking steps to develop terminator crops that render themselves sterile after one growing season. The losers will be farmers who will find themselves beholden to the seed makers every growing season.[18]

Genetic modification of food is intrinsically dangerous, as it involves making irreversible changes to DNA structures that we still do not yet fully understand (and maybe never will), despite great advances made by the Human Genome Project. It is inevitable that this will lead to a disaster.

Obesity

Obesity is epidemic on a global scale.

This did not occur overnight. It has become more and more of an issue over the past 50 years, slowly increasing at first, and then escalating over the past couple of decades. In the United States, in the year 2000, 67.5% of men and 57.5% of women were overweight or obese.[19]

Genetic factors and/or some illnesses can cause obesity, but by far the main cause is diet and lifestyle. Obesity primarily has two causes: overeating and lack of exercise. Although you cannot change your genetic makeup, you can control eating habits and levels of activity.

In the western world, the choice of processed foods has increased dramatically. Supermarkets stock thousands of line items giving a far greater selection of products than any time in the past. Pre-packaged foods, fast-food restaurants and cafes are now available with such abundance, with calorie overdosing now endemic.

Portion sizes are increasing as well, with the marketing term super-size now common. The National Institute of Health calls this "portion distortion," and has compared foods today against 20 years ago by average portion size...[20]

Food	Calories 20 Years Ago	Calories Today
Bagel	140	350
Cheeseburger	330	590
Spaghetti & meatballs	500	1,025
Soda	85	250
French fries	210	610
Turkey sandwich	320	820
Blueberry muffin	210	500
Pizza slices (2)	500	850
Popcorn	270	630
Chocolate chip cookies	55	275

Obesity and overweight is measured by using the Body Mass Index (BMI). This is a measurement of weight divided by the square of a person's height. For example, an 80kg person who is 1.8 meters tall has a BMI of $80 / 1.8^2 = 24.7$. The following shows accepted ranges for BMI...

BMI Value Range	Description
Under 19	Underweight
Between 19 and 25	Normal weight
Between 25 and 30	Overweight

Between 30 and 35	Obese
Over 35	Morbidly Obese

There really is no specific ideal weight, as there are many factors involved. For example, it is possible for a healthy, muscular individual with low body fat to be classified as overweight or obese using the BMI formula. What the BMI does do, however, is provide a guide to a healthy range of weight for average individuals.

Childhood obesity is of particular concern, with some one in ten children being obese. The worldwide problem of childhood obesity is recognized and described as follows...[21]

> *Obesity is set to become the biggest disease of the century. Health experts say that curbing childhood obesity could prevent millions of cancer cases and other illnesses. Childhood and adolescent obesity occurs when a child has too much body fat. Obesity is usually caused by both overeating energy-dense nutrient-poor foods and a lack of exercise. Levels of childhood obesity are increasing at alarming rates in many countries including the United States, the United Kingdom and Australia. [Better Health Channel]*

Obesity also reduces our life span, and for the first time in 1,000 years, life expectancy is expected to decrease. We are literally eating ourselves to an early death.[22]

Failure of Diets

Diets all essentially rely on one factor: severe calorie intake reduction. While calorie reduction to base levels is a good practice, excessive reduction does not achieve the desired result due to built-in calorie deprivation mechanisms. Firstly, excessive lowering of calories does not help the body burn off fat. Instead, the body reduces its level of metabolism in what it interprets as being a period of starvation, and consequently attempts to hold on to whatever fat reserves it has. Since the body is in preservation mode, low calorie diets deplete us of energy and make us feel tired and lethargic. To counter inadequate intake of nutrients and minerals, many diets recommend the use of supplements. These are, however, very poor substitutes for obtaining all our nutrients from food, are often very expensive and made of dubious ingredients.

Many who have tried various calorie-restricting diets end up binge eating then putting back on the weight they lost - yo-yo dieting. Not only are these diets ineffective, but they also add to the sense of frustration and failure when lower weights cannot be maintained. In a nutshell, diets are…

Too High In Fat: Even so-called low fat diets can be too high in fat. Many commercial diet plans are still around 25% of calories from fat because they still permit consumption of meat, dairy products and eggs.[23] In order to reduce meals down to 300 or 500 calories, there is no choice but to reduce the volume of food.

Boring, Bland & Unimaginative: Dry crackers with a slice of cheese and celery stick each day for lunch just does not do it!

Too Difficult: Many diets require meticulous calorie counting and restriction, portion sizing, complex exchanges and endless journaling. It all gets too hard!

Use Wrong Foods: Many diets contain the wrong foods, or rely on dietary supplements, food substitutes, pills and other questionable concoctions. High protein, low carbohydrate diets are not only ineffective, but are quite dangerous.

The feeling of persistent hunger is as uncomfortable as it is unnatural. You find yourself hanging out to eat your next meager portion and in the end give up in frustration, followed by a sense of guilt and remorse over your "lack of willpower." After depriving the body of calories, as soon as an opportunity to eat presents itself, the all too familiar binge occurs. This is often followed by a sense of guilt and failure, even depression. Worse still, the weight just comes right back on again.

Fad Diets

There is seemingly no end to the number of fad diets available today. Generally, they can be identified by applying the following checks: Do they claim to lose weight rapidly? Do they claim that you can lose weight and keep it off without giving up fatty foods? Do they advocate that exercise is not an important factor, or do they neglect exercise? Do they market their plan with fancy books, packages, pre-prepared foods, pills, elixirs and other concoctions? Do they charge an arm and a leg for these? Do they require you to eat specific foods on a continuous basis, such as cabbage soup, every day?

The Atkin's Diet is singled out here because of its high popularity and complete anti-thesis of the vegetarian Genesis diet. This fad diet is comprised mainly of meats, chicken, cheese, eggs, butters and oils with no limit. It follows a series of phases, the first being the Induction phase that lasts for 2 weeks. The next phase of the diet plan, the Maintenance phase, is less restrictive by allowing some vegetables and raising carbohydrate levels slightly.[24]

The theory behind the low-carbohydrate Atkins diet is that the body must turn to fat and protein as sources of energy. When energy is obtained this way, ketone levels in the blood and urine increase, a condition known as ketosis.[25] This is a similar condition to that of uncontrolled diabetes.

Health issues from following the Atkins diet include increased risk of colon cancer, increased risk of cardiovascular and heart disease, impaired kidney function, bone-calcium loss, constipation, dehydration, bad breath and general tiredness.[26]

One such health issue befell Florida businessman Jody Goran. Mr Goran went on the Atkins diet at the age of 50 for 2½ years. He is now suing Atkins Nutritionals arguing that the Atkins diet caused him to develop severe coronary disease, elevated cholesterol levels, angina pains, and a blocking of arteries requiring an angioplasty and a stent. He is seeking only $15,000 damages, saying that his real intention for filing the lawsuit was to raise public awareness and warn about the potential dangers of the Atkins diet.[27]

Food Guide Pyramid

The well known Food Guide Pyramid found on most food packaging had its origin in 1894 when the US Department of Agriculture (USDA) published its first dietary guidelines for the American nation. These recommendations included 5 food groups: dairy, meat, fruits and vegetables, fats and fatty foods, sugar and sugary foods.[28]

In 1941, a National Nutrition Conference was called into action by President Franklin Roosevelt. As a result of this conference, Recommended Daily Allowances (RDA's) were presented for Americans to follow, and in 1943, the

Basic Seven nutritional guidelines were developed to deal with food shortages during World War II. These seven groups were later reduced to four basic groups: dairy, meats, fruits and vegetables, and grain products. Even so, due to the increase in diseases like stroke and heart disease, a fifth group, fats, sweets and alcohol, was added in the 1970's to ensure that these were eaten in moderation.[29]

The USDA's food guide was published annually, however, many did not know it existed. So in 1992 the Food Guide Pyramid was introduced in graphic style in an attempt to convey recommended proportionality of consumption. Those foods at the bottom of the pyramid were to be consumed in greater quantities than those at the top.[30]

So concerned that the Food Guide Pyramid does not reflect the healthiest diet possible, the Harvard School of Public Health issued the following statement...[31]

> *The information embodied in this pyramid doesn't point the way to healthy eating. Why not? Its blueprint was based on shaky scientific evidence, and it hasn't appreciably changed over the years to reflect major advances in our understanding of the connection between diet and health. [Harvard School of Public Health]*

Nutritionists today recognize many flaws in the Food Guide Pyramid, and its recommendations have generated quite a lot of controversy. Much debate centers on whether the Food Guide Pyramid has been influenced by agricultural interest groups such as the dairy and meat industries. Another criticism is that the pyramid lumps together both plant and animals sources of protein and therefore treats them equally.[32]

All this points to the fact that building an acceptable

food pyramid is a very difficult, if not impossible, thing to do. Firstly, there is the interests and intense lobbying of large and powerful agricultural industries. Secondly, there is the false premise that animal products should be consumed daily for good health. And thirdly, the notion that dairy products are required for calcium is so prevalent (but nonetheless wrong), it would be a brave move to exclude them.

On April 19, 2005, the USDA released a new food guide replacing the Food Guide Pyramid. The new system, called MyPyramid, provides twelve separate food guides depending on daily calorie requirements.[33] It also encourages regular physical activity. However, do not be fooled. The meat, livestock, dairy and processed food industries are very powerful and have lots of money. They will continue to lobby to ensure that their products are well represented in any national food recommendations.

New Four Food Groups

In order to present an alternative to the flawed Food Pyramid, the New Four Food Groups was proposed in 1991 by Dr Neal Barnard, MD, president of the Physicians Committee for Responsible Medicine (PCRM).[34] These new four food groups are FRUITS, VEGETABLES, LEGUMES and WHOLE GRAINS, at the exclusion of all animal products. Dr Barnard states…[35]

> *What is most noteworthy, of course, is that two of the old food groups — meat and dairy — have been dropped: Meats — all meats, poultry, and fish — contain cholesterol and saturated fat, and all meats are totally devoid of fiber and contain virtually no complex carbohydrates. So there is no meat*

group in the New Four Food Groups. Like-wise, dairy products contain fat, cholesterol, lactose, and allergenic proteins, and have no fiber or complex carbohydrates. So there is no longer any recommendation that dairy products be included in the diet. [Dr Neal Barnard]

Botanically speaking, it can be difficult to strictly classify plant foods, just as it is difficult to taxonomically categorize animals. For example, herbs do not sit well as they are loosely defined as plants or parts of plants that are valued for their medicinal, savory or aromatic properties. Herbs could be given their own, fifth classification. However, for simplicity and in line with the general understanding of what constitutes a fruit or vegetable, the New Four Food Groups provides an excellent basis for food classification with respect to the Genesis Diet.

Fruits
Fruits are the edible, pulpy, ripened ovaries of flowers from plants such as trees and vines. Fruits bear within them mature seeds for propagation of the plant. In Genesis 1:29, it is defined as the fruit that yields seed. Many foods considered vegetables are in fact fruit, such as tomatoes, cucumbers, pumpkins, squash and peppers.

Vegetables
Vegetables are the edible part of plants that are not regarded as a fruit. In common usage, vegetables include stems (celery, rhubarb), leaves (lettuce, spinach), roots or tubers (potatoes, radish, carrots), bulbs (onions, leeks) and flowers (broccoli, asparagus). Fungus plants such as mushrooms are also regarded as vegetables.

Legumes

Legumes are plants that have seeds in a pod, such as beans, peas, chickpeas, peanuts and lentils (from the Latin word for lens indicating the shape of a lentil). Rich in proteins, carbohydrates, B vitamins, iron and minerals such as potassium, magnesium, iron and zinc, legumes are inexpensive powerhouses of nutrition.[36] They form an important part of the diet of many peoples around the world, however, they are often neglected in our western diet. The small quantity of fat in legume is mostly unsaturated, but does not contain any cholesterol to clog up arteries.

Probably one of the best-known legume is the soybean. Henry Ford, during the Great Depression of the 1930's, used soybean oils to make automotive enamel paints and soybean meal converted to plastic to make car parts such as horn buttons and gear shift knobs. Henry Ford's scientists also invented soybean wool and Ford himself wore suits made from soybean fiber.[37]

Although soybeans are not generally eaten as beans in their own right, they are processed into many different products, both edible and non-edible. These include traditional foods such as tofu, tempeh and soy sauce, and today, soybeans are made into dairy product substitutes (such as milk, cheese, yogurt, cream, butter, whipped toppings and infant formulas), flour, textured protein, substitute meat analogs, and non-dairy frozen desserts. Needless to say, the fat contents of these substitute foods need to be examined carefully.

Whole Grains

Grains include wheat, oats, corn, rice, millet, barley and seeds, as well as products made from them such as bread, pasta and cereals. Grains and seeds are matured, fertilized ovules (the structure of the plant containing the female egg cell) generally associated with grasses. They contain lots of fiber, complex carbohydrates, proteins and minerals, and no cholesterol.

Acid/Alkaline Balance

The term pH refers to the "power of hydrogen" or the "potential of hydrogen." Mathematically, $pH = -\log_{10}[H+]$, that is, minus log to the base 10 of the concentration of H+ ions in solution. This translates to a scale of 1 to 14, with pH of 7 being neutral, neither alkaline nor acidic. Acids have pH levels less than 7 while Alkalines (also known as Bases) have pH levels greater than 7. The closer to pH of 7, the weaker an acid or alkaline is.[38] Acids easily form with alkalines to produce salt and water.

The precision at which the pH level of the blood and extracellular fluid is maintained is of extreme importance. Other fluids, such as urine, saliva and stomach acids can tolerate a wider range of pH, but the blood is maintained within a very narrow range. Dr Joel Robbins, MD, DC, a popular speaker on health issues, says this about the pH levels maintained in the body…[39]

> *Our internal body chemistry functions in an alkaline environment. Our blood must maintain a pH of 7.4. If it drops below that to 7.2 we die. The cells of the body in health are alkaline. In disease the cell pH is below 7.0. The more acid the cells become, the sicker we are and feel. The cells won't die until their pH gets to about 3.5. Our bodies produce acid as a by-product of normal metabolism. This is the result of our bodies burning or using alkaline to remain alive. Since our bodies do not manufacture alkaline, we must supply the alkaline from an outside source to keep us from becoming acid and dying. [Dr Joel Robbins]*

Since pH levels are logarithmic, a decrease in pH value of 1 means a 10-fold increase in acidity. For example, an acid that has a pH of 4 is ten times more acidic that an acid with pH of 5. Similarly, an alkaline with pH of 9 is ten times more alkaline than an alkaline with pH of 8. Thus, a change in pH of just 0.2 means a change of 1.58 times ($10^{0.2} = 1.58$).

Of most importance, particularly over the long-term, is the acid/alkaline balance of food. In the digestive process, the acid/alkaline balance is affected by the secretions of acids from the stomach and bicarbonates from the pancreas. After eating, there is a temporary change in blood pH levels that quickly returns back to optimal pH levels. However, sustained and excessive consumption of acid-forming foods does not readily allow the body to revert back to correct pH levels.

As a general rule, animal foods, fats, oils, legumes and grains/nuts/seeds are acidic, while fruits and vegetables are alkaline. The standard western diet is far too high in fat and protein from excessive consumption of animal products, producing a constant state of high acid toxicity, or acidosis.

Common alkaline and acid foods include...

Alkaline Foods: All fruits and vegetables, some nuts (almonds, chestnuts) and seeds, herbal and green teas, spices and peppers. Even citrus fruits such as oranges and limes are alkaline when digested due to organic citrates that are metabolized into alkaline bicarbonates.

Acidic Foods: All fats and oils, all grains (except millet, which is alkaline), all dairy products, nuts (cashews, brazil, peanuts, pecans, walnuts), animal meats (fish, chicken, pork, beef), pastas, alcohol, beans and legumes.

A diet high in fruits and vegetables is in harmony with

the body's own acid/alkaline balance. Plant based acid foods, such as grains, should still be incorporated, firstly to avoid excessive alkalinity but also to obtain many essential plant nutrients and fiber. Generally speaking, acid/alkaline foods should be consumed in a ratio of 80% alkaline and 20% acidic.[40] This rule is easily achieved on the Genesis Diet. A diet rich in meats, fats, dairy and eggs tips the acid/alkaline balance too far in the acidic direction.

Powerful Protection

Smoke, pollution, automotive emissions, carbon monoxide, pesticides, herbicides, fertilizers, heavy metals, solvents, chemical food additives and inorganic minerals all infiltrate our bodies in the air we breathe and the food we eat. They wreak their destructive havoc in our bodies. In addition, there are internally produced toxins caused by the metabolism of foods and other bodily processes.

Every second of every day, there is a battle against these toxins and the destructive unstable free radicals they produce. Free radicals are formed when damage is caused to the intricate chemical balance by pulling electrons out of their normal orbits. This causes an instability or possible chain reaction when liberated electrons send free radicals into the bloodstream.[41]

Fatty cell membranes, called lipids, wrap each cell of the body, however, free radicals can penetrate these membranes eventually damaging cells and their internal structures. Unabated free radical attack can result in damaged cell machinery giving rise to renegade cells that multiply without control, causing tumors and cancers.[42]

Free radicals are combated by antioxidants such as carotenoids, flavonoids, selenium and vitamin E. All these protective phytonutrients (plant nutrients) are found in plant foods that constitute the Genesis Diet. Continued sustenance of these foods provides us with a consistent source of protection against disease-causing free radicals.

Carotenoids

During the bleak days of 1941, when England stood alone against the Luftwaffe, outstanding pilots such as John Cunningham, a leading night fighter pilot, chalked up 20 kills. He was nicknamed Cats' Eyes, and his exceptional skill was said to be because he ate lots of carrots to improve his night vision.[43] This rumor was spread to mask the fact that England had radar technology. From that time on, mothers have encouraged their children to eat their carrots, quite a good thing to do.

Carotenoids are fat-soluble pigments found principally in plants. There are currently over six hundred known carotenoids, of which some 50 have vitamin A precursor potential.[44] One such carotenoid is beta-carotene, a potent antioxidant found in copious amounts in yellow and orange vegetables such as carrots, sweet potatoes, pumpkins and squash. Beta-carotene serves as a powerful biological antioxidant, protecting cells from the damaging effects of free radicals and oxidation. Other functions include enhancement of the immune system, protection from sunburn and inhibition of the development of some cancers.

Beta-carotenes pass from the plasma into the eye, and along with vitamin C and E, provides substantial protection against cataracts and macular degeneration.[45] So while carrots don't make humans see in the dark, they do provide large amounts of beta-carotene that help us maintain good eyesight.

Flavonoids

First identified in the 1930's by Albert Szent-Gyorgyi, the Nobel laureate who discovered vitamin C, flavonoids were originally referred to as vitamin P.[46] Szent-Gyorgyi found that two flavonoids derived from citrus fruit decreased capillary fragility and permeability. However, the chemical diversity of flavonoids precludes them from being classified as a single vitamin.

Flavonoids are found in the pigments of fruits and vegetables, giving them their fantastic array of rich colors. The brilliant oranges in carrots, the bright reds in tomatoes, the luscious blues and purples in berries, grapes and cherries all get their vibrant colors from flavonoids contained within them. A visit to the market or greengrocer reveals wonderful arrays of beautiful and vivid colors found in displays of fruits and vegetables. Some five thousand different flavonoids are currently identified.[47]

Most flavonoids have anti-inflammatory, anti-viral and anti-cancer forming properties. They are also powerful antioxidants, just like their carotenoid cousins. A high dietary intake of fruits and vegetables is consistently associated with reduced risk of cancers including lung, breast, prostrate and colon cancer.[48]

Minerals

Although minerals do not provide energy (which can only be obtained from the metabolism of carbohydrates), they are essential for good health. Minerals work in combination with each other and other nutrients, so imbalances can lead to health problems.

Some important minerals include…

Calcium (Ca): The most common mineral in the body, with 98% contained within the bones and the remainder circulating in the blood and taking part in metabolic processes. Vegetarian foods high in calcium include soy and rice milks, tofu and tempeh, leafy green vegetables, beans, nuts, dried figs, tahini, broccoli, etc.[49]

Chromium (Cr): Works with insulin to utilize blood glucose and controls metabolism of triglycerides.

Copper (Cu): Critical in the absorption of zinc and iron.

Iodine (I): Essential to the functioning of the thyroid gland.

Iron (Fe): Aids in red blood cell generation and prevents anemia.

Magnesium (Mg): Magnesium is essential for maintaining the acid-alkaline balance in the body, as well as healthy functioning of the nerves, muscles and cardiovascular system.

Manganese (Mn): Necessary for normal bone formation and important enzyme reactions.

Molybdenum (Mo): Involved in the operation of key enzymes.

Phosphorous (P): Assists in food metabolism and aids the self-repair of body tissues.

Potassium (K): Along with Sodium, Potassium is a primary regulator of fluids inside cells, and is critical in the transmission of nerve cells, muscle contraction and blood pressure. Fruits and vegetables are rich in potassium.

Selenium (Se): A trace mineral required only in very small quantities but is essential to good health. The mechanism by which selenium exerts its beneficial effects on health is through proteins containing selenium, known as selenoproteins. The antioxidant properties of selenoproteins help prevent cellular damage from free radical attack. While selenium can be found in some animal foods, plant foods are the major dietary source. However, concentrations of selenium depend on the amount of selenium contained in the soil, which can vary from place to place. Grains and nuts are particularly rich in selenium.

Zinc (Zn): Supports the health of the immune system and governs the contractility of muscles.

Vitamins

Vitamins were first discovered by the Dutch physician, Christiaan Eijkmann, who won the Nobel Prize for medicine in 1929.[50] Vitamins are essential for good health and perform many critical functions, including regulating metabolism and assisting biochemical processes that release energy from digested foods. They protect health by boosting the immune system, and aid in the formation of hormones, blood cells and nervous system transmitters. They also act as catalysts for hundreds of important chemical reactions in the body.

Supplements can be beneficial in certain situations, however, it is far better to obtain vitamins through eating plant foods. The exception to this rule is Vitamin B_{12}, which is the only vitamin that cannot be obtained from plant sources, and therefore when on the Genesis Diet, should be supplemented daily, either from fortified foods such as soymilk, or direct supplementation from tablets.

The following is a summary of currently known vitamins...

Vitamin A: Derived from carotene, a vitamin

precursor found in fruits and vegetables. It affects the formation of skin, mucous membranes, bones, teeth, vision and reproduction.

Vitamin B: Actually a complex of a number of different essential chemicals. These work together to bolster metabolism, maintain healthy skin, enhance immune and nervous system function, and promote cell division. The B vitamins include Thiamine (B_1), Riboflavin (B_2), Niacin (B_3), Pantothenic Acid (B_5), Pyroxidine (B_6), Biotin (B_7), Folic Acid (B_9) and Cobalamin (B_{12}).

Vitamin C: Ascorbic Acid is a well-known vitamin. It assists in the formation of collagen and plays a major role in the formation of bones and teeth. It also enhances the absorption of iron from vegetables.

Vitamin D: This vitamin is necessary for the formation and retention of calcium and phosphorous in the bones. Vitamin D is manufactured in the body when sterols migrate to the skin and become irradiated with sunlight. Vitamin D is the only vitamin that can be manufactured in the body.

Vitamin E: Vitamin E is a fat-soluble vitamin that exists in eight different forms. A powerful antioxidant, vitamin E is found in the natural oils of grains, nuts, fruits and leafy green vegetables. It is delivered to each cell via the bloodstream where it positions itself in the cell membrane waiting to neutralize free radical attacks. Oxidative changes to LDL cholesterol ("bad" cholesterol) promote blockages in the coronary arteries, which ultimately lead to pains in the chest (angina) and heart attack. By limiting the

LDL cholesterol oxidation, Vitamin E plays a role in protection against cardiovascular and heart disease.

Vitamin K: This vitamin is required for coagulation of blood.

Carbohydrates

There are two major carbohydrate classifications: simple and complex.

Simple Carbohydrates contain one or two sugar molecules known as monosaccharides and dissacharides respectively. Refined, simple carbohydrates such as table sugar and products made from them (lollies, candy bars, etc) are highly concentrated carbohydrates stripped of any nutritional benefit. Consuming sugar creates a burden on the pancreas and over-production of insulin, causing fluctuations in blood glucose levels. Foods containing highly processed simple carbohydrates should be avoided.

Complex Carbohydrates contain three or more sugar molecules, otherwise known as polysaccharides, which include starches, glycogen and fiber. These must be pulled apart during digestion. This process takes a considerable amount of time thereby releasing sugars more slowly into the bloodstream at an optimal rate (particularly important for diabetics).

The most powerful weight-control menu is a vegetarian one. Plant foods, particularly in their raw and unprocessed state, are rich in complex carbohydrates but low in calories. Fruits, vegetables, legumes and whole grains are the indisputable master foods for energy and weight reduction.

It is a myth that carbohydrates, such as potatoes, are fattening (it is not the potato that is fattening, but the cheese with sour cream topping). Carbohydrates signal your brain to switch off your appetite when you have had enough to eat and increase your metabolism by activating thyroid hormones circulating in the blood.

Fiber

Dietary fiber is an important and essential component of our daily food intake. Only plants contain fiber, while animal foods such as meat, dairy products and eggs contain none.[51] The modern western diet, based primarily on animal products and processed foods, is very deficient in fiber and is a factor in the onset of many degenerative diseases, particularly colon cancer.

There are two main categories of fiber: soluble and insoluble.[52] Soluble fiber dissolves in water forming a jelly like substance (as occurs when cooking oats), while insoluble fiber (cellulose) cannot be digested. Since high-fiber foods are bulkier and need to be chewed, the body's satiety triggers are more effective, reducing the chance of overeating. Chewing also stimulates the production of saliva where enzymes begin the first stage of digestion.

Dr Norman Walker, DSc, who studied the science of nutrition for many years, wrote about the importance of fiber to our health…[53]

> *The fiber which is so essential for the proper and complete digestion of our food is needed in the colon just as much as in the small intestine. Such fiber, however, must be composed of roughage, that which is found in raw foods. When these fibers pass through the intestines they become, figuratively speaking, highly magnetized, and in this condition are very helpful in the functions involved in the various parts of the intestines. In addition to receiving the residue of that part of our food that is not digested, the colon also accommodates itself*

*to the fiber — the roughage — in the food
upon which it depends for its "intestinal
broom." [Dr Norman Walker]*

Fiber assists in bulking up stools in the colon and minimizes their transit time. If there is insufficient fiber, stools become hard and dry. These tend to stick to the walls of the colon reducing its ability to absorb spent material for elimination and allow toxins in the feces to be reabsorbed back into the body. As years pass by, the accumulation of fecal material narrows the colon causing disturbed bowel movements such as constipation, diarrhea and irritable bowel syndrome. Continuous straining pressure by the muscles that push feces through the colon causes the development of hernias, varicose veins (due to pressure on the veins of the legs), hiatus hernia (upward pressure of the stomach into the chest), diverticulitis (weakening and infection of the colon wall) and anal hemorrhoids. Colorectal cancers are more common in people who have had lifelong constipation problems due to the concentrated exposure of carcinogens in the colon.[54]

Fat and Cholesterol

Fats are compounds containing long chains of carbon atoms with oxygen and hydrogen atoms attached to these chains. These molecular chains contain constituent fatty acids, and collectively, fats, oils and fatty acids are known as lipids.

There are different types of fats, depending on their carbon-hydrogen bond makeup...

Saturated: Every available carbon bond contains a hydrogen atom, that is, saturated with hydrogen. Saturated fats are solid at room temperature, like lard or butter. Saturated fats are derived from animals and are always associated with high levels of cholesterol.

Unsaturated: Not all available carbon bonds contain hydrogen atoms. Unsaturated fats are liquid at room temperature, like olive oil. Unsaturated fats are primarily derived from plant sources and do not contain any cholesterol.

Monounsaturated: Like unsaturated fat, but one pair of carbon atoms in the chain share a double bond rather than a single bond.

Polyunsaturated: Also like unsaturated fat, but two or more carbon atom pairs contain a double bond.

Partially Hydrogenated: These are unsaturated fats that have been made saturated by heat or other chemical means. Margarine is a prime example of a partially hydrogenated fat.

Omega-3 and Omega-6: Both are essential polyun-saturated fatty acids, since they must be obtained from food. While it is true that fish and fish oils provide copious amounts of these fatty acids, eating fish is not recommended due to the high protein and cholesterol levels associated with the flesh. Plant sources rich in omega-3's and 6's are nuts (walnuts, brazil nuts, hazelnuts), sesame seeds, chick peas (and humus dip made from chick peas), and leafy green vegetables.

Cholesterol has a lot of stigma attached to it, but it provides vital functions such as making cell membranes, producing hormones and making bile acids. It also acts as a transport medium for moving fatty acids through the bloodstream.[55]

Cholesterol is not really a fat, but more like a waxy substance primarily manufactured in sufficient quantities by the liver, thus dietary intake of cholesterol is not required. The problem occurs when excess cholesterol is obtained through foods. Once inside the body, dietary cholesterol finds itself in the bloodstream where it will be deposited in the tissues and on the walls of arteries. No plant food contains cholesterol, including oils produced from plants, such as grapeseed or olive oil.

The fat you eat is the fat you wear.[56] This is true for all types of fats and oils, so while using olive oil is better than butter, all fats and oils should be kept to a minimum. Fat is inefficiently digested and is not the body's primary source of energy fuel. Fat does not have the metabolism boosting effects that carbohydrates do. Each gram of fat contains 9 calories, while each gram of protein and carbohydrate contains only 4.[57] Fat, in all its forms, is a calorie dense food.

When all types of fat are eaten, bile acids secreted into the stomach break it down into more digestible particles. These particles find their way into the bloodstream causing the blood to become thicker and stickier. This reduces blood circulation and consequently causes a drop in oxygen supply to the cells of the body.

Dr John McDougall, MD, describes the horrors of this process...[58]

> *Blood cells within the blood vessels flow freely and bounce off one another prior to a high-fat meal. Approximately one hour after a fatty meal, the cells begin to stick together on contact and form clumps. As this clump formation progresses, the flow of blood slows. Six hours after the meal, the clumping becomes so severe that blood flow actually*

stops in many small vessels. Several hours later the clumps begin to break up and the blood flow returns to the tissues. As a result of these changes, the oxygen content of the blood decreases by 20 percent. The consequences of this impaired circulation can be angina, impaired brain function, high blood pressure, fatigue, as well as compromise of the function of any other body part. [Dr John McDougall]

For this reason, meals containing moderate or high levels of fat are not recommended to people diagnosed with heart disease, where even a single fatty meal can cause the onset of angina pectoris due to oxygen deprivation of the coronary arteries. With a few exceptions (such as avocados and olives), fruits and vegetables have very little fat (and no cholesterol).

A comparison between animal and plant foods shows no contest for fat and cholesterol levels...

Animal Foods	**Fat(gm)**	**Cholesterol(mg)**
Full cream milk (1 cup)	10	30
Cheddar cheese (30gm)	10	30
Butter (1 tablespoon)	16	45
Whole egg	6	210
Beef steak (120gm)	12	100
Chicken drumstick	7	85
Tuna in brine (100gm)	3	40

Plant Foods	**Fat(gm)**	**Cholesterol(mg)**
Tofu (100gm)	5	0
Rice (100gm)	1	0
Wholemeal bread (1 slice)	1	0
Vegetables (100gm)	0 to 2	0

Nuts and seeds (50gm)	10 to 30	0
Fruit	0	0
Olives (ten)	2	0

In the western world, we are eating too much fat, but particularly saturated animal fats. Fat, particularly in excess, is a burden to our bodies that we do not need, and we must eliminate it from our diets for efficient weight loss and good health maintenance.

Some fat is essential for good health, and it cannot be avoided entirely anyway. Nuts, seeds and grains contain certain amounts of fat, however, as we have seen, we should not consume more than 10% of calories from fat, and only from unsaturated sources. For example, if your daily calories are 2500 then the maximum calories from fat are 250, giving a fat allowance of nearly 30 grams per day. Note also that oils are liquid fat, and therefore must be included in this amount. All animal fats should be avoided, but of course, to do this, all animal foods must be avoided.

And the fat of a beast that dies naturally, and the fat of what is torn by wild animals, may be used in any other way, but you shall by no means eat it. Leviticus 7:24

Beware of hidden sources of fat, even in vegetarian foods. Always look out for the fat content in foods. For example, potato crisps are 30% fat and contain a lot of unhelpful salt! When you eat meat (red, white, poultry and fish), you are eating the fat and stored calories of an animal. Even if you cut external fat off, the so-called lean meat itself is still marbled with it, and still yields high amounts of calories from fat. Moreover, cholesterol is primarily found in the lean portion of meat.[59]

Protein

Amino acid units form the structure of all proteins and DNA and therefore form the building blocks of all life. Of the eighty or so amino acids currently identified, twenty are necessary for growth and repair. Of these twenty amino acids, eight are called "essential" because they need to be obtained from food, while the remainder are manufactured in our bodies.[60]

Not every individual plant food contains all twenty amino acids, but all twenty amino acids are obtained from a balanced plant-based Genesis diet. It was once considered necessary to combine certain plant food groups together in the same meal, for example, grains and beans, however, more recent research indicates that this is not required.[61] Provided a plant-based diet consists of a range of servings from the New Four Food Groups, all necessary amino acids and proteins will be obtained, but without the harmful fat and cholesterol.

Although animal proteins and plant proteins are built from the same amino acids, their structures are quite different. Animal proteins tend to be higher in sulfur compounds that cause a drop in pH levels to more acidic levels. The idea that animal proteins are superior to plant proteins is bunkum.

Our protein needs are actually quite low, certainly no more than 10% by calories. John Robbins, director of EarthSave and author of Diet for A New America, examined the issue of protein requirements, and reported...[62]

> *I've had to wonder whether we might have been misled about our protein needs. Feeling a little unsure, I've turned to the light of recent unbiased scientific research, to get a better understanding of what our protein needs might be. These are studies produced by groups without a product to sell. I've*

> *found that not all authorities agree on a precise figure for our daily needs of protein, but their calculations do fall within a specific range. It is a range that runs from a low esti-mate of $2\frac{1}{2}$% of our total calories up to a high estimate of over 8% [John Robbins]*

At this low level, it is impossible not to consume enough protein on the Genesis Diet. As a percentage of calories, plant foods are higher in protein than many realize. Legumes are, of course, well known to be high in proteins, even comparable to meat, however, grains, fruits, vegetables, nuts and seeds also supply adequate amounts.

The following table shows percentages of calories from protein for a range of vegetarian foods...[63]

Legumes	Percentage
Soybean sprouts	54%
Tofu	43%
Green peas	30%
Lentils	29%
Split peas	28%
Kidney, navy and lima beans	26%

Grains	Percentage
Rye	20%
Wheat	17%
Wild rice	15%
Oatmeal	12%
Barley	11%
Brown rice	8%

Vegetables	Percentage
Spinach	49%
Kale, broccoli	45%

Brussel sprouts	44%
Cauliflower	40%
Lettuce	34%
Zucchini	28%
Cucumber	24%
Peppers, artichokes, cabbage	22%
Eggplant	21%
Tomatoes	18%
Potatoes	11%

Fruit	**Percentage**
Lemons	16%
Honeydew	10%
Cantaloupe	9%
Strawberries, oranges grapes	8%
Watermelon	8%
Peach	6%
Pear, banana, grapefruit	5%

Nuts & Seeds	**Percentage**
Peanuts	18%
Walnuts	13%
Cashews	12%

Excess protein consumption is dangerous, as would be the case in a diet containing animal foods. Such excessive amounts of protein forces the liver and kidneys into overload, and for this reason, people with kidney diseases are instructed to keep meat and other animal foods to a minimum (of course, it would be far better to remove them from the diet entirely).

Based on a very generous 10% of calories from protein, a male who eats 2500 calories per day requires only about 60 grams of protein, while a female on 2,000 calories requires only 50. Compare this with the amount of protein for a typical day on a meat-based western diet...

Breakfast

2 eggs (60gm each)	20 gm
2 slices toast with butter	13 gm

Lunch

Ham, cheese and tomato sandwich

Ham (30 gm)	6 gm
Cheese (30 gm)	10 gm
Tomato	1 gm
White Roll	7 gm

Snack

Chocolate bar (150 gm)	8 gm

Dinner

Meat and veggies

Steak (400 gm)	116 gm
Veggies (300 gm)	3 gm
Sauce	1 gm

Snack

Sweet biscuits (100gm)	11 gm
Total:	***188 gm***

This example shows a total protein intake some three or four times the daily recommended allowance!

Osteoporosis

Osteoporosis is a condition whereby the amount of bone material decreases in quantity and quality over time. Bone mass becomes more and more porous and thinner, making the bones more brittle and susceptible to fractures. The architectural integrity of the skeleton begins to decrease, particularly in the spine causing stooping and other deformities. It is often called the "silent disease" because bone loss occurs over a long period of time with no symptoms.

Hips are particularly susceptible to fractures due to osteoporosis, hence the hip fracture incidence (that is, the number of hip fracture cases per 100,000 person-years) is used as a measurement of osteoporosis in a given population.

Dairy Products No Protection

It is often feared that removal of dairy products from the diet will lead to a calcium deficiency, and therefore give rise to osteoporosis. The Dairy industry understands and promotes this fear by constantly advertising the "need" to consume three servings of dairy per day.[64] This is enough to keep the profits rolling in, but does not sound too excessive as to seem irresponsible.

Far from being beneficial, however, the consumption of dairy products actually increases the risk of osteoporosis despite the quantities of calcium found in dairy products. This may seem like a fantastic statement, however, the evidence is that there is a definite relationship between dairy consumption and hip fracture incidences (HFI). Professor Jane Plant has this to say about this relationship...[65]

> *The marketing of dairy produce as an essential source of calcium has been so strong that even some medical professionals, who should know better, insist that eliminating dairy produce from the diet will lead to calcium deficiency and hence increase the risk of osteoporosis. In this book, we present evidence, from peer-reviewed scientific literature, which strongly and convincingly refutes this. Indeed, we believe that we show that this is one of the great myths of our time.*

> *... We have researched the subject further and found compelling evidence in the scientific literature that it is the Western diet and lifestyle that is the root of the problem. Far from being beneficial, the consumption of dairy products, especially cheese, is actually damaging to those at risk of osteoporosis and other bone diseases. **For many people, cheese is likely to be part of the cause, not the cure, of osteoporosis** (emphasis, theirs).*
> *[Professor Jane Plant]*

The following table shows average milk consumption per person per year versus hip fracture incidence...[66, 67]

Country	Dairy Intake(kg)	HFI
Finland	370	140
Sweden	341	200
The Netherlands	329	130
France	256	100
United States of America	254	160
Italy	239	130
Australia	233	120
New Zealand	210	120
Kuwait	177	120
Spain	164	80
Chile	120	20
Venezuala	96	40
Gambia	17	10
China	8	60

Clearly, it can be seen that there is a strong correlation between higher dairy intake and osteoporosis as measured by hip fracture incidence. So then, the question must be asked: Why is the incidence of osteoporosis higher in countries where dairy consumption is high? The inescapable conclusion is that dairy is a factor in the onset of osteoporosis (as we have previously discussed), a conclusion that the dairy industry certainly does not like.

What About Calcium?

Understandably, when dairy products are removed from the diet, the nagging question is always "Where do I get my calcium?" Before answering this question, it is interesting to note some pertinent points in relation to dairy consumption.

For a start, humans are the only "animals" to consume milk when weaned, and are the only "animals" that drink the milk of other animals. Once a baby is weaned off milk, there is no further requirement for milk protein. Most adults cannot digest lactose (milk sugar) because they no longer produce the lactate enzyme necessary for milk metabolism. This is known as lactose intolerance.[68]

Milk is pasteurised at very high temperatures effectively destroying any nutrients contained therein. And milk is actually a high fat food, too. In terms of percentage of calories by fat, milk measures in at nearly 50 percent! This is because milk contains about 90% water, which has no calories. There are up to 4.6 billion fat globules per millilitre of milk.[69]

African Bantu women, who live mainly on a vegetarian diet and eating very little animal food, including dairy, have a calcium intake of only 300 to 400 mg per day. This compares to the recommended daily allowance of 1200 mg specified by health authorities in western countries.[70] Yet these women have many children and breast-feed them until they are weaned. They do not have calcium deficiencies and osteoporosis is rare among them. How can these women achieve this amazing feat with such a low intake of calcium?

Adequate amounts of calcium are easily obtainable in the Genesis diet. There are many alternatives to dairy for obtaining healthy amounts of calcium, such as leafy green vegetables, broccoli, squash, sweet potatoes, legumes, chickpeas, soybeans, tofu, nuts, (almonds, hazelnuts and walnuts), and dried fruits, particularly figs. All fruits and vegetables contain some calcium, and they have the benefit of a myriad of other vitamins, minerals and nutrients, as well as plenty of fiber.

The problem with milk is that it is mainly a protein, and all proteins, particularly animal proteins, form an acidic ash when digested. This causes the bloodstream to acidify, and therefore calcium is readily extracted from the bones to correct the blood's pH level. Blood calcium levels clearly take priority over bone calcium levels in the economy of calcium distribution and pH correction.

Thus, calcium loss is not an issue of insufficient calcium intake, but rather maintaining calcium balance within the body. Even with very high calcium intakes of up to 1400 mg per day, if the diet is high in animal proteins, there will still be a net loss of calcium from the bones.[71]

Heart Disease, Stroke & Atherosclerosis

Atherosclerosis is a condition whereby the arteries carrying life-giving blood begin to harden and narrow. This process can start very early in childhood, where fatty streaks are deposited in the inner walls of the arteries. These fatty streaks build up over time into unstable plaques, which often rupture causing deadly blood clots known as thrombotic occlusions.

Blood that passes through the chambers of the heart does not nourish the heart itself. Rather, the heart is supplied by the coronary arteries, so called because they form a corona around the heart. Partial deprivation of oxygen to the heart due to thrombotic occlusions is known as angina pectoris, which is accompanied by very acute pain. It is a severe warning that serious arterial blockage is present in the coronary arteries.

If the arterial blockage occurs in the arteries to the heart, a myocardial infarction (heart attack) occurs as the heart muscles are starved of oxygen. Similarly, a stroke is caused by blockages in the arteries to the brain, and the brain is deprived of oxygen.

Reversing Heart Disease

The very notion that heart disease could be reversed was previously thought to be impossible. Even up to a couple of decades ago, the idea that diet and lifestyle could reverse heart disease was only a radical concept. It was always believed that there was nothing people in the real world could do about it.

Dr Dean Ornish, MD, a pioneer in heart disease prevention using diet and other lifestyle principles, has developed heart disease prevention and reversal dietary plans based on vegetarian foods. Dr Ornish states...[72]

> *In general, the more cholesterol and fat you eat, the higher will be your blood cholesterol level and your blood pressure. High blood cholesterol levels and high blood pressure increase the risk of coronary heart disease. The more cholesterol and saturated fat you eat, the greater your risk of coronary heart disease, even if your blood cholesterol level and blood pressure do not rise very much. People who eat a low fat, low cholesterol vegetarian diet ... have low blood pressure and low blood cholesterol levels in childhood that remain low as they get older, and they have very low rates of coronary heart disease. People who eat a typical American diet have low blood pressure and low cholesterol levels*

*in childhood that tend to increase as they get
older, and they have high rates of coronary
heart disease. [Dr Dean Ornish]*

The Genesis Diet, based solely on plant foods, will ensure
that the intake of dietary fat and cholesterol levels will significantly decrease, allowing the process of plaque formation to
reverse. This will initially take the tension off plaque
surfaces, and then allow the plaques to decrease in size.

Dr John McDougall, MD, another pioneer in the application of diet to reverse heart disease, says this about animal
foods in relation to heart disease...[73]

*Avoid all foods of animal origin, including
the following: red meat, poultry, fish,
seafood, eggs, milk, butter, cheese, yogurt,
and sour cream. These foods contain
extremely high quantities of fat and cholesterol. In fact, animal products are the primary
source of saturated fat and cholesterol.
Saturated fat dramatically raises blood
cholesterol levels and leads to atherosclerosis and heart disease. All forms of fat
increase your chance of contracting diabetes,
cancer, obesity, and other degenerative
diseases. [Dr John McDougall]*

Framingham Heart Study

The Framingham Heart Study has involved the residents
of Framingham, Massachussetts, for over 50 years. It is the
longest running clinical study in medical history. It follows a
representative sample of 5,209 adult residents and their
offspring (the Offspring Study). The study's goal is to determine circumstances under which cardiovascular and coronary
heart diseases occur. With data collected over these 50 years,

some 1,000 scientific papers have been written identifying major risk factors of heart disease, stroke and other diseases.[74]

Before the study, doctors believed that atherosclerosis (hardening of the arteries) was an inevitable part of the aging process and blood pressure was supposed to increase with age. This is because they did not understand that there was a relationship between high levels of cholesterol and heart disease, and there was no recognition that modification of eating habits could avoid or reverse these diseases.

According to the Framingham Heart Study web site...[75]

> *Since its inception in 1948, the Framingham Study has had a profound effect on our understanding of the major risk factors associated with developing heart and vascular disease and stroke. Perhaps as important, the work has stimulated numerous national awareness campaigns educating the American public to the "heart risks" tied to untreated high blood pressure and high cholesterol levels and the dangers of smoking. And, the study has played a seminal role in influencing physicians to place greater emphasis on prevention and detecting and treating cardio-vascular disease risk factors in their earliest stages. [Framingham Heart Study]*

Dr William Castelli, MD, director of the Framingham Heart Study, concludes by saying, "Vegetarians have the best diet. They have the lowest rates of coronary disease of any group in the country. Some people scoff at vegetarians, but they have a fraction of our heart attack rate and they have only 40 percent of our cancer rate. They outlive other men by about six years now."[76]

Cancer

The word cancer itself comes from the Latin word for crab because the swollen veins around a tumor appear like the legs of a crab.

A fundamental characteristic of cells is their ability to reproduce themselves by dividing, a process known as mitosis. This process is well regulated, however, if cells begin to multiply in a haphazard and uncontrolled manner, the result is a cumulative mass of non-structured material referred to as a tumor. Cancer cells can also spread to other parts of the body through the bloodstream and lymphatic system.[77]

Although cancer in children account for only 0.3% of all cancers, it is the second greatest killer of children under 14.[78]

Toxic Load

In our modern world, carcinogenic pollutants bombard us daily and increase the toxic load in our bodies. Such pollutants include auto exhaust, industrial and agricultural pollution, cigarette smoke and radiation. Pesticides, herbicides, fungicides and other chemicals find their way into our food supply, ready to wreak chemical havoc.

Dr Don Colbert, MD, a Christian medical doctor specializing in the area of toxicity and fasting, has this to say about toxins...[79]

> *Every day we are exposed to thousands of toxins, and they are slowly accumulating in our bodies. If we do not get toxic relief, these poisons may eventually kill us through sickness and disease. [Dr Don Colbert]*

Carcinogenic carbon compounds are created when meats are cooked, causing further toxicity when metabolized. All these factors conspire to create a poisonous environment in our bodies. Therefore, it is of utmost importance to minimize exposure to this toxic load as much as possible.

Our bodies need to be cleaned of dangerous and damaging garbage on a constant basis. In simple terms, cancer occurs because the body has more toxins than it is capable of processing. In this state, cellular damage begins to accumulate, and eventually becomes serious, if not irreversible, unless harsh measures are taken.[80]

Cancer Protection

By far, the best "cure" for cancer is not to get it in the first place, and the body is well designed and capable of preventing and crushing malignancies. However, it needs to be given sufficient arsenal to do the job.

By giving immune cells the ammunition they need, they will be able to perform their task efficiently. They are willing to kill and be killed for the sake of continued good health and protection. A healthy immune system not only protects against all manner of foreign and threatening chemicals, but also seeks out and destroys mutinous cancer cells, an activity that goes on every minute of every day of our lives.[81] Plant foods, particularly in their raw, natural state, contain nutrients that assist in the continuous battle against toxicity, free radical activity, and cancer formation.[82]

As much as eighty percent of cancers are due to factors that are individually controllable. Of these factors, up to 50% of cancers are attributed to poor diet, such as that which is typically eaten in the western world.[83] The following percentages apply for cases of cancers that can be prevented by eating a high intake of fruits and vegetables and avoidance of animal foods...[84]

Cancer	Percentage
Breast	33 to 50%
Uterine	25 to 50%

Cervix	25 to 50%
Prostate	40%
Lung	20 to 33%*
Colorectal	10 to 20%

* Smoking remains the major cause of lung cancer.

It is encouraging that cancer councils and societies around the world are beginning to recognize the link between diet, obesity and cancer. The American Cancer Society states...[85]

Eating right, being active, and maintaining a healthy weight, are important ways to reduce your risk of cancer—as well as heart disease and diabetes. Eat five or more servings of a variety of vegetables and fruits each day. Choose whole grains in preference to processed (refined) grains and sugars. Limit consumption of red meats, especially those high in fat and processed. Choose foods that maintain a healthful weight. More than a decade ago the National Cancer Institute launched the Eat 5 A Day for Good Health program to move Americans closer to a cancer-fighting diet. Today the evidence is even stronger that a diet high in fruits and vegetables can help prevent cancer over a lifetime. [American Cancer Society]

Diabetes Mellitus

All sugars and starches are broken down by the digestive system into a simple sugar called glucose, which is the energy food for every cell in the body. Glucose is transported by the blood and escorted into each cell by insulin. If there is insufficient or no insulin, or insulin is unable to perform its duty satisfactorily, glucose levels in the blood begin to rise (hyperglycemia), causing the condition we know as diabetes.[86] In effect, diabetes is starvation of the cells for the food (glucose) they need. This is why diabetics often feel very tired and sleepy.

Left unchecked, diabetes leads to many health maladies such as thirst, dehydration, tiredness, poor blood circulation (often leading to limb amputation), blindness due to damage to delicate retinal blood vessels, and kidney failure. It is potentially the fastest growing disease in the western world.

Many diabetics need daily injections of insulin, as well as the constant need to prick their fingers to measure their blood glucose levels. The constant juggling of insulin and eating can create a roller-coaster ride of high and low sugar levels. Low sugar levels (hypoglycemia) can result in coma or even death.

In the United States in 2002, approximately 18.2 million people had diabetes. The total estimated cost of the disease was $132 billion — about 1 out of every 10 health care dollars spent.[87] Diabetes is the 6th highest cause of death.[88]

There are three major types of diabetes…[89]

Type 1: The inability of the pancreas to produce insulin or enough insulin. This type of diabetes often strikes early in life and is sometimes referred to as juvenile diabetes.

Type 2: A condition where insulin is being produced by the pancreas, but is unable to efficiently escort glucose into the cells.

Gestational Diabetes: Occurs in pregnant women, however, this condition is mostly alleviated when birth occurs. Nevertheless, women who experience high levels of gestational diabetes need to be monitored to ensure this does not develop into other types of diabetes.

Eating too much refined sugar is indeed unhealthy, and places a burden on the liver and pancreas, as well as causing fluctuations in blood sugar levels. However, sugar is not actually the primary cause of diabetes. Rather, it is the high fat, high protein diet typically eaten in the western world...[90]

> *Sugar is not the cause of Type 1 or Type 2 diabetes. People with diabetes do have to be careful with sugar because their bodies do not deal with it well. But the primary culprit in diabetes is not the sugar. For Type 2 diabetes, it's the fat-rich, animal-protein-rich, super-serving-sized eating pattern that too many of us have become accustomed to. This overly fatty diet causes us to gain weight, clogs our arteries, pushes our blood pressure up, and encourages our cells to become insulin-resistant. For many, Type 2 diabetes follows. [Physicians Committee for Responsible Medicine]*

Diabetic societies and councils around the world do, of course, recognize that diet and exercise are major factors in the control of the disease. However, they seem to be reluctant to be drawn into the issue of whether a pure vegetarian diet is appropriate for diabetics, instead preferring to remain with the standard diet defined by the Food Guide Pyramid. The American Diabetes Association unfortunately advises diabetics to base their meals on the Food Guide Pyramid that still allows meat, dairy and eggs to be eaten.[91]

This unfortunately ignores the power of a vegan diet like the Genesis Diet to control and reverse diabetes. The very low fat level in the Genesis Diet ensures that insulin is allowed to do its job with minimal hindrance. The complex carbohydrates and fiber found in plant foods regulate a slower release of sugars into the bloodstream.

According to Dr Neal Barnard, MD...[92]

> *In study after study, scientists have found that diets high in fiber-rich foods — fruits, vegetables, beans and whole grains — reduce the risk of diabetes. [Physician's Committee for Responsible Medicine]*

A high complex carbohydrate, low-fat diet encourages weight loss, which is good news for diabetics. Complications from the disease are significantly lower when a more healthy weight is maintained.

Pharmaceuticals

Hard-working doctors, nurses and hospital management have to constantly make decisions in the face of overwhelming numbers of people presenting with all manner of diseases and health maladies.

For example, Jack is 42 years old and has not exercised for years. He has become overweight and decides to go running in a futile effort to reduce weight. All of a sudden, Jack collapses with a heart attack, and fortunately for him, some other joggers see him, perform CPR and call an ambulance. While in the ambulance, paramedics literally bring him back from death. After two weeks stay in the hospital, he is allowed to go home. Jack is a "lucky" man, but his life will never be the same again.

The paramedics, doctors and nurses involved in Jack's

case are to be congratulated for picking up the final pieces of a long history of physical neglect and ignorance. Could Jack have avoided this episode in the first place?

Jill finds herself tired all the time and she too has put on quite a few extra kilograms. She is constantly thirsty and has to urinate all the time. A visit to her local doctor shows that her blood sugar levels are way too high and so she is sent to the hospital. In the hospital, Jill is given insulin injections and is subjected to all sorts of tests. Finally, after a few days, her blood sugar levels begin to reduce and she finds that the dryness in her mouth begins to abate, but she is informed that there has been significant damage to her kidneys.

The doctors and all those involved in Jill's case are to be congratulated for picking up the final pieces of a long history of physical neglect and ignorance. Could Jill have avoided this episode in the first place?

These stories are fictional, but certainly not atypical. Jack and Jill's stories are repeated in almost every hospital in the country, every day.

All this is not to say that there is nothing to criticize in modern medical practice. Drugs are often inappropriately prescribed, incorrectly dosed, their side effects not fully understood or they are simply ineffective. One particular example is the overuse of antibiotics, the most widely prescribed drug in the western world...[93]

> *Antibiotics are often prescribed "just in case" to people not in hospital. They cannot cure the common cold or other viral infections such as influenza, but they are often given "just in case" a bacterial infection gets a foothold. Antibiotics should never be given "just in case," and they are not suitable for self-limiting illnesses such as colds and flu. [David Jackson and Rayner Soothill]*

Of course, not all drugs are evil, and not all are useless. They can often be life saving, however, we should do all we can to minimize, if not eliminate, the use and dependency on drugs.

US Senate hearings in the early 1960's brought in a wave of laws and regulations relating to the approval and marketing of drugs. Today, despite understandable protestation from the pharmaceutical industry, clinical proof that a drug is effective is required before it is approved for marketing. Such regulation has at least provided some level of protection for the end-user.

Nevertheless, the use of drugs to treat illness and disease is increasing at an alarming rate, further adding to the cost of health. Is this use (or over-use) of drugs resulting in a healthier population? Indeed, prescription medications, while important for treating some medical conditions, is the cause of more than 1 million hospitalizations in the United States annually. The over-use of medications is rampant.[94]

Needless to say, the production of drugs is now a huge, multi-billion dollar industry, and like all big business, there is concern for the bottom line. As a result, the pharmaceutical industry spends huge amounts on self-promotion. In 2001, spending in the United States was estimated at $12.5 billion after the Food and Drug Administration (FDA) relaxed rules on direct-to-consumer advertising.[95]

Dr Randall Stafford, MD, assistant professor of medicine at the Stanford Prevention Research Center, says this about how marketing affects a medical practice...[96]

> *Our findings suggest a complex relationship between marketing, scientific evidence and prescribing patterns. Physicians should recognize that the promotion of pharmaceuticals might have a bigger impact on their practice than they often acknowledge,*

> *particularly when evidence is lacking. [Dr*
> *Randall Stafford]*

How can it be that the medical establishment, from universities, clinics and hospitals be overly influenced by the pharmaceutical and food industries? Although there are independent scientific researchers doing research on a number of diseases, particularly in the relationship between food and disease, they do not have any real voice in the current establishment. It is difficult for them to get their results published in scientific journals. Generally, the cashed up pharmaceutical and food industries perform their own 'research', which can hardly be accepted as totally unbiased.

Dr Jay Cohen, MD, describes drug company shenanigans like this...[97]

> *Aggressive marketing, slanting research, unethical publishing of results, pressuring medical centers, intimidating researchers, influencing physicians, limiting information, manipulating the FDA, marketing drugs with inaccurate safety information and inappropriate doses — all of these have created an environment in which medication development has become a "race to the bottom." [Dr Jay Cohen]*

Not only are there issues with prescription drugs, but also an increasing number of non-prescription over-the-counter drugs are available to anybody who wants to buy them. Further added to this are thousands of so-called natural health products available in health stores, supermarkets or from individuals involved in network marketing schemes. There appears to be no requirement for these products to pass clinical proving trials that at least the pharmaceutical companies are required to do.

Another huge problem is the drug-dependency culture of the western world. This dependency can range from prescription drugs, over-the-counter drugs (eg, pain killers), illicit narcotics and legal drugs such as alcohol, nicotine and caffeine. There are literally hundreds of commonly abused drugs, with the most-abused drugs being cocaine, marijuana and heroin. This is followed by anti-anxiety drugs, tranquilizers and sedatives (amphetamine, diazepam such as valium, methamphetamine such as 'speed', methadone), cough medicines and hallucinogenics such as lysergic acid (otherwise known as LSD or 'acid').[98]

Food as Medicine

Regarded as the father of modern medicine, Hippocrates lived in the fifth century BC. He was born in the island of Cos, and belonged to the family that claimed to be descendents of the mythical Aesculapius, son of Apollo. Hippocrates' works include some of the earliest extant Greek medical writings, including the famous Hippocratic Oath.

Hippocrates is famous for coining the phrase "Let food be your medicine and medicine be your food," and he compiled a list of some 400 herbs and their uses. The use of natural medicine from nature dates back thousands of years through many different cultures, from the bizarre to those that clearly work.

Although it is proven that food plays a major role in the development of sickness, very little time, if any, is actually dedicated to the study of food and its relation to disease in medical learning institutions. Worse still, any education and information regarding food supplied to doctors and hospitals are supplied by the food industries. I remember seeing in the hospital waiting room posters telling us that we should get our "three servings of dairy." But guess where these posters came from? Yes, the dairy industry!

In today's modern western medical practice, medicine being food and food being medicine is given scant regard, although this is changing slowly. The last decade has seen a resurgence of interest in the use of plant foods for medicinal purposes. This interest may be due to inadequate treatment of chronic conditions, and perceived shortcomings of conventional health care.

Many foods and spices are prized in other cultures for their medicinal properties. Garlic, ginger, cumin and tumeric, for example, are common throughout Asian and Eastern countries, so it is fortunate for western societies that migration and cross-cultural mingling has introduced these foods more and more to the dinner table.

The following is a sample of beneficial foods that have medicinal properties.

Aloe Vera comes from the Arabic word Aloeh meaning "shining bitter substance." Native to Africa, the gel from the aloe vera plant and crystalline part found along the leaf blade are both used for medicinal and topical purposes, particularly wounds and burns, where it is capable of speeding up the repair of damaged skin. It is also a valuable topical treatment for skin conditions such as eczema, itchy skin (urticaria), dermatitis and acne rosacea. The aloin found in aloe vera acts as a gentle laxative, assisting the passage of stools through the intestines.

Bananas are an excellent energy food because they contain three forms of sugar: fructose, glucose and sucrose. Combined with fiber, bananas provide a consistent, sustained source of energy. It is therefore the number one fruit with leading athletes.

Due to their very high potassium levels, bananas combat anemia by stimulating hemoglobin production in the blood. This makes them the perfect food to combat high blood pressure. So effective are bananas in reducing blood pressure the

US Food and Drug Administration has given the banana industry permission to make official claims regarding the fruit's ability to reduce the risk of blood pressure, heart attack and stroke.[99]

Broccoli contains many disease fighters and includes antioxidants that are high in cancer fighting activity. Like most cruciferous vegetables, it speeds up removal of estrogen thereby suppressing breast cancer. Broccoli is also a high source of chromium to help regulate insulin and blood sugar levels.[100]

Garlic has been used for thousands of years for various purposes, from maintaining health to repelling demons and vampires! Such association with superstition and folk medicine may be one reason why garlic has not taken its rightful position as a medicinal herb.

Written accounts of garlic as an herbal and medicinal remedy date back thousands of years. When Moses led the Isrealites through the wilderness, they reminisced of the food they ate in Egypt, such as cucumbers, melons, leeks, onions, and garlic. (Numbers 11:5). During World War 1, doctors successfully treated gangrene with the juice of garlic known as "Russian penicillin."

It is now known that garlic regulates blood lipids such as cholesterol, triglycerides and other fat molecules. Lower cholesterol levels substantially reduce the risk of cardiovascular and heart disease.

Garlic helps to fight allergies such as hay fever, neutralize heavy metals such as lead, mercury, copper, silver and aluminum, and assists in the prevention of cancer by stimulating the body's immune system.

While garlic may not ward off vampires, in terms of being a cancer fighter, it is the general leading the army to battle. Benjamin Lau, MD, PhD, professor of immunology and microbiology, School of Medicine, Loma Linda University, has this to say about garlic's cancer fighting properties...[101]

> *Garlic apparently stimulates the body's immune system, particularly enhancing the macrophages and lymphocytes, which destroy cancer cells. [Dr Benjamin Lau]*

The active ingredient in garlic is allium sativum. It is rich in vitamin B_1, an enzyme used in carbohydrate metabolism that keeps the nerves of the body healthy. It also contains vitamins A and C, and is a good source of minerals. Garlic has enormous powers to fight parasite infections in the gastronintestinal tract, and also kills bacteria, yeast and virus. [102]

Ginger is believed to have originated in India. It is a perennial herb containing underground branch roots called rhizomes. It has a characteristic odor when cut. Ginger was introduced to China at a very early date, where it has been used as a medicine and spice ever since.

Both fresh and dried ginger contains effective herbal and medicinal value. While the plant is not really palatable on its own, it is often cooked into recipes giving them wonderful and unique flavors.

Ginger has always been used as a medicinal plant for digestive disorders dyspepsia, flatulence, colic and spasms and other afflictions of the stomach and bowels. It also acts as a pain killer in arthritic and musculoskeletal disorders.

Capsaicin, a crystalline alkaloid, is the substance that gives capsicums, chilies and peppers their pungency.

Pure extracted capsaicin is actually so potent that chemists handling it must work in filtered rooms in full body protection. It is believed that capsaicin is a secondary metabolite, a chemical that is not required to support the life of the plant, but rather fights off animal predators. For example, it has been observed that animals to not eat chilies, but birds do, allowing the seeds to be spread far and wide.

More importantly, capsaicin acts as an anti-inflammatory agent and helps to control pain. It is a natural painkiller, and acts by blocking the transmission of pain signals to the brain. Other benefits of capsaicin may be to assist digestion by stimulating the flow of saliva and stomach secretions, and an anti-microbial to help control infections such as pneumonia.[103]

Spinach and other green, leafy foods may help reduce the risk of macular degenerative disease (the macula, the part of the retina at the back of the eye, allows our eyes to focus on fine details), which is a gradual, painless deterioration of the macula, but leaves peripheral vision intact. The two active ingredients are lutein and zeaxanthin, which give these vegetables their deep green color. These phytonutrients counteract the damage of free radicals in the macula.[104]

Tomatoes contain lycopene, which becomes more available to the body after tomatoes are heated, such as in canned tomatoes and tomato sauces. Increased consumption of lycopene has been associated with reduced risk of cancer of the prostate, breast, digestive tract, cervix, bladder, and skin.[105]

Chapter 3
GOING VEGETARIAN

Without doubt, God's original diet for mankind is a plant food regimen.

> **And God said, See, I have given you every herb that yields seed which is on the face of all the earth, and every tree whose fruit yields seed; to you it shall be for food. Genesis 1:29**

The psalmist recognized the importance of a vegetarian diet...

> **He causes the grass to grow for the cattle, and vegetation for the service of man, that he may bring forth food from the earth. Psalm 104:14**

Some of the reasons you may decide to adopt this diet are that it is God's original diet to man, is the healthiest diet available and matches the low-fat, high fiber diet recommended by many dieticians and doctors, and has the ability to reverse diseases such as heart disease and diabetes. Additional reasons may be objections to cruelty meted out to factory farmed animals, disapproval of killing animals and concern for the environment and the world's resources.

The American Dietetic Association, in a position paper regarding vegetarian diets, confirms the effectiveness of vegetarian diets in fighting disease...[1]

> *It is the position of the American Dietetic Association and Dietitians of Canada that appropriately planned vegetarian diets are healthful, nutritionally adequate, and provide health benefits in the prevention and treatment of certain diseases. Interest in vegetarianism appears to be increasing, with many restaurants and college foodservices offering vegetarian meals routinely. Substantial growth in sales of foods attractive to vegetarians has occurred, and these foods appear in many supermarkets. Vegetarian diets offer a number of advantages, including lower levels of saturated fat, cholesterol, and animal protein and higher levels of carbohydrates, fiber, magnesium, boron, folate, antioxidants such as vitamins C and E, carotenoids, and phytochemicals. [American Dietetic Association]*

Ultimately, however, it is a highly personal and individual decision to make. It is hoped that this book provides an insight into the Biblical approach to nutrition, what God's ideal diet is and what it can do for you.

In Good Company

King Nebuchadnezzar, having just conquered the fortified city of Jerusalem, spoke an edict that only the most impeccable young individuals, including certain Jews, were to be taught and trained three years for the highly responsible vocation of serving in his palace. They were to eat the same diet as the king, probably containing foods offered to Babylonian gods.

> **So Daniel said to the steward whom the chief of the eunuchs had set over Daniel, Hananiah, Mishael and Azaria, Please test your servants for ten days, and let them give us vegetables to eat and water to drink. Then let our countenances be examined before you, and the countenances of the young men who eat the portion of the king's delicacies; and as you see fit, so deal with your servants. So he consented with them in this matter, and tested them 10 days. And at the end of ten days, their countenance appeared better and fatter in flesh than all the young men who ate the portion of the king's delicacies. Daniel 1:11-15**

Although all the candidates were already "without blemish or physical defect," after the 10 days were over, Daniel was even healthier and better nourished than those who ate the king's food. What a testimony to the wisdom of God who created man to be vegetarian. Daniel knew the secret to health, well-being and longevity of life.

Another interesting aspect to this passage of scripture is Daniel's use of the scientific method thousands of years before being formally devised in the 16th century by Francis Bacon. Stressing experimentation, observation, measurement and induction from data rather than philosophical musings, it is accepted practice in today's world to perform controlled experiments where one group is subject to special conditions and compared to another control group maintaining the status quo. At the end of the experiment, changes to the subject group are compared to the control group and the results collated and analyzed.

Needless to say, Daniel's experiment proved highly

successful and he was allowed to continue to eat his vegetables and drink water for at least the remainder of his training.

Many Christian leaders were vegetarians. One of the earliest Christian documents is the Clementine Homiles, a second century work reputedly based on teachings by Peter the Apostle. The author, St Clement of Alexandria, wrote...

> *It is far better to be happy than to have your bodies act as graveyards for animals. Accordingly, the apostle Matthew partook of seeds, nuts and vegetables, without flesh. [St Clement of Alexandria]*

Saint Basil, otherwise known as Basil the Great, was born in Caesarea in 329AD. Though born of noble stock, Basil was renowned for organizing famine relief and working in the kitchen himself, something nobles would not have done. Being a very popular speaker, and fearful that he would be puffed up with pride, Basil sold all he had and became a priest. He fought Arianism, a heresy that denied the divinity of Jesus. St Basil wrote...

> *The steam of meat meals darkens the spirit. One can hardly have virtue if one enjoys meat meals and feasts. In the earthly paradise there was no wine, no one sacrificed animals, and no one ate meat. [St Basil]*

St Jerome, born in 340AD, owes his place in history for his exegetical studies and translations of the Bible. In particular, he translated the Latin Bible still in use today. As for eating animal flesh, St Jerome did not hold back his words...

> *The eating of meat was unknown up to the big*

flood, but since the flood they have the strings and stinking juices of animal meat into our mouths, just as they threw in front of the grumbling sensual people in the desert. Jesus Christ, who appeared when the time had been fulfilled, has again joined the end with the beginning, so that it is no longer allowed for us to eat animal meat. [St Jerome]

Born in 1182, Francis of Assisi was a Roman Catholic saint who took the Bible literally. His humble following grew into the Franciscan Order. St Francis is revered as the Patron Saint of Animals, and once even preached to sparrows! His devotion to the love of animals and man reflects the Lord's compassion to all his creation.

The Lord is Good to all, and His tender mercies are over all His works. Psalm 145:9

On animal cruelty, St Francis exhorted...

All things of creation are children of the Father and thus brothers of man, God wants us to help animals, if they need help. Every creature in distress has the same right to be protected. If you have men who will exclude any of God's creatures from the shelter of compassion and pity, you will have men who deal likewise with their fellow men. Not to hurt our humble brethren is our first duty to them, but to stop there is not enough. We have a higher mission - to be of service to them wherever they require it. [St Francis]

Modern western vegetarianism is derived mainly from Christian roots. John Wesley was an Anglican clergyman, who along with his brother Charles, organized a Bible study group at Oxford. The group soon became known as Methodists because of their emphasis on methodical study and devotion. Wesley rejoiced that...

> *Thanks be to God! Since the time I gave up the use of flesh-meats and wine, I have been delivered from all physical ills. [John Wesley]*

He further taught that animals...

> *...shall receive ample amends for all their present sufferings. [John Wesley]*

In 1809, the Reverend William Cowherd established the Bible Christian Church, in which members of the congregation had to take a vow not to eat meat. The Bible Christian Church provided leadership of the Vegetarian Society in England and helped found the International Vegetarian Society. The Reverend William Metcalfe left England with a group of pilgrims from the Bible Christian Church and set up a branch in Philadelphia, from which the American Vegetarian Society was formed.[2]

William and Catherine Booth devoted their lives to serving the poor in London when, in 1864, William began open-air meetings with drums and musical instruments. They also started a Christian Mission, which later became the Salvation Army.[3] On eating animal flesh, William Booth had this to say...

> *It is a great delusion to suppose that flesh-meat of any kind is essential to health. Considerably more than three parts of the work in the world is done by men who never*

taste anything but vegetable, farinaceous food, and that of the simplest kind. There are more strength-producing properties in wholemeal flour, peas, beans, lentils, oatmeal, roots, and other vegetables of the same class, than there are beef or mutton, poultry or fish, or animal food of any description whatever. [William Booth]

In a passionate plea to Christian leaders regarding cruelty to animals, Catherine Booth exhorted...

The awful cruelty and terror to which tens of thousands of animals killed for human food are subjected in traveling long distances by ship and rail and road to the slaughter-houses of the world. God disapproves of all cruelty, whether to man or beast. The occupation of slaughtering animals is brutalizing to those who are required to do the work.... I believe this matter is well worthy of the serious consideration of Christian leaders. [Catherine Booth]

Many influential Christians in the 19th and 20th centuries laid the foundations of modern Christian vegetarianism. Even back in the 1850's ordained ministers, such as Sylvester Graham of the Presbyterian Church, organized a convention that marked the beginning of the Vegetarian Movement in America. In the 19th century, many ministers lectured on vegetarianism and health, as well as why Christians should reject the killing and eating of animals.[4]

Even Theodore "Teddy" Roosevelt supposedly threw his breakfast sausages out the White House window after reading Upton Sinclair's book The Jungle that exposed corruption and abuses in the meatpacking industry at the turn of century.[5]

Unfortunately, today, there is virtually no mention of man's cruelty to animals from the pulpit of mainstream churches.

Famous Vegetarians

Many famous people are vegetarians or vegans, including Christian leaders past and present, as we have seen. Only a few are listed here, however, much more comprehensive lists are readily available on the Internet. See also Appendix C for a sample of quotations by a number of vegetarians.

Albert Einstein (scientist): Famous mathematician and theoretical scientist who devised the General Theory of Relativity and awarded a Nobel Prize for physics in 1921.

Benjamin Franklin (US statesman, inventor): Inventor of the Franklin heat efficient stove and bifocal glasses. He worked on the committee that drafted the American Declaration of Independence and a signatory to the Constitution.

Christian Barnard (surgeon): Performed the first open heart transplant in history.

Isaac Newton (scientist): Sir Isaac Newton is famous for formulating the law of universal gravitation, determining laws of motion and kinematics, developing calculus, laws of energy conservation and the particle theory of light. He also constructed the first reflecting telescope. What is not well known about Newton is that he was a genuine Christian and wrote many books and articles defending the faith, refuting atheism, defending the Ussher chronology and upholding the creation account in the Bible.

Leonardo da Vinci (scientist, artist, inventor): One the best known figures of the Renaissance. Gifted with a curiosity of the physical world, he explored geology, botany, hydraulics, aeronautics, mechanics, anatomy — the list goes on.

Pythagoras (mathematician): Described as the first pure mathematician. The Theorem of Pythagoras states that the square of the hypotenuse of a right-angled triangle is equal to the sum of the squares of the other two sides.

Film and TV Personalities: Pamela Anderson, Bridgette Bardot, Kim Basinger, Alec Baldwin, Drew Barrymore, Candice Bergen, Carol Burnett, Leonard di Caprio, Dan Castellanata (voice of Homer Simpson), John Cleese, Billy Connolly, Penelope Cruz, Ted Danson, Doris Day, Danny DeVito, Clint Eastwood, Michael J. Fox, Dustin Hoffman, Richard Gere, Gerrard Kennedy, Ricki Lake, Spike Milligan, Demi Moore, Paul Newman, Guy Pearce, Brad Pitt, Jerry Seinfeld, Peter Sellers, William Shatner, Brook Shields, Lynda Stoner, Mr T, Mary Tyler-Moore, Dennis Weaver, Kate Winslet.

Popstars and Musicians: Shirley Bassey, Kate Bush, Bob Dylan, George Harrison, Whitney Houston, B52s, Billy Idol, Davy Jones, John & Yoko Lennon, Paul & Linda McCartney, James McCartney, Don McClean, Meatloaf (strange name for a vegetarian!),

Olivia Newton John, Ringo and Barbara Starr, Tina Turner, Richard Wagner.

Sports Men and Women: Peter Brock (car racing), Chris Campbell (champion wrestler), Greg Chappell (cricket), Robert De Costella (marathon runner), Cory Everson (Ms Olympia 6 times), Ruth Heidrich (ironwoman), Billy Jean King (tennis), Bruce Lee (martial arts), Carl Lewis (track and field), Edwin Moses (athletics, 8 gold Olympic medals), Martina Navratilova (tennis), Murray Rose (swimmer, 3 Olympic gold medals), Bill Pearl (Mr Universe), Gary Player (golf), Dave Scott (Ironman triathlon), Serena Williams (tennis).

Philosophers, Artists, Writers, Inventors: Susan Anthony (leader of women's sufferance movement), Aristotle, Confucius, Thomas Edison, Ghandi, Steve Jobs (founder of Apple Computers), Plato, Plutarch, George Bernard Shaw, Albert Shweitzer (humanitarian), Socrates, Leo Tolstoy, Mark Twain, H. G. Wells.

Geoffrey Giuliano, an early Ronald McDonald clown, threw in his rubber nose, striped socks and yellow suit to become a vegetarian. He repented of his years of "deceiving thousands of innocent, trusting children" while working for "the McDonalds corporate juggernaut," as well as being ashamed of his stint performing children's magic shows for the Burger King Corporation.[6] Giuliano's tenure at McDonalds included a $50,000 annual salary (not bad for 1978), a private chef, limo service and a personal secretary. In an effort to make amends for past sins, Giuliano is developing a magic show he plans to take to schools and vegetarian food fairs. He added, "This show is my way of saying sorry for selling out so blatantly to concerns that make their millions off the murder of countless animals and the exploitation of children for their own ends."

Transitioning to a Vegetarian Diet

Go all the way! Do not tease yourself by eliminating some foods here and some foods there. Smokers who go cold turkey have the greatest success rate in giving up the habit. The same applies with giving up animal products.

Start by throwing out all foods of animal origin from your refrigerator and pantry. This includes meat, milk, ice-cream, eggs, yogurts, butters, etc. That may be a lot of food, but don't worry about it, you are on a very important journey (maybe you could give your meat to the neighbor's dog, who is far better designed to deal with it!) Remember, you are throwing out stuff that is quite harmful to your health. If it's not in the house, then you can't eat it.

Cook yourself a delicious vegetarian meal that you may already eat without thinking about it. Maybe you like to eat spaghetti with bolognaise sauce and some side salad. Well, this time, simply substitute the bolognaise sauce with a delicious tomato Neapolitan sauce. Add as much delicious salad as you like. If you like burritos, why not use chili beans instead of meat?

Then go to the supermarket and restock your kitchen. Now that you have decided not to eat animal products, you'll probably find that 80% of the supermarket is of no use to you — definitely makes shopping easier! In time, you will learn to shop for vegetarian only foods — it's all part of your new adventure. While you're out shopping, buy yourself one or two good vegetarian (or better, vegan) cookbooks to inspire you.

Adopting new menus and cooking methods is easier than you may think, and it can be exciting as you explore new ways to prepare meals. Your journey may take you to many local and exotic locations, such as India with its traditional vegetarian cuisine spanning more than two millennia. There are hundreds of wonderful Indian vegetarian recipes such as Dal Makha (lentils with onions, tomatoes, ginger, garlic and spices), Chana Masala (chick peas cooked with spices), Rajma (kidney beans cooked in onion tomato gravy and spices), Aloo Matar (potatoes and peas cooked in tomato sauce and seasonings), and many, many more.

How about sensational Asian rice, noodle, vegetable, stir-fry, bean curd and tofu dishes? There are wonderful Italian pasta and spaghetti recipes. Head south of the border to Mexico for delicious burritos, chili bean recipes, tomato salsas, guacamole and tacos. From Africa come delicious Moroccan salads, bean soups, lentil soups, vegetable stews and Ethiopian breads. And from Greece and the Middle East we get wonderful tobouli salads, falafels, hummus dips, dolmas (stuffed grape leaves), kebabs, Lebanese and pita breads. The list of international and traditional vegetarian recipes is huge. And the beauty of most of these recipes is that they are relatively easy to prepare.

It is important to include the whole family in your journey. If they are prepared to join you, then you are home and hosed. If other members of the family do not wish to join in with you, at least come to some arrangement — they will not try to talk you out of it and you will not veggie-bash them! They will soon start to take notice when they see you slimming down, becoming more active and looking much better! Your actions and results will speak far louder than any words.

And through all this, be absolutely confident in what you are doing. If you have read this book, it is my prayer that the arguments presented here make sense to you. But don't just stop here. Read and learn as much as you can, and when you have finished, read some more! Filling your head with knowledge helps you to combat doubts, helps you to resist contrary opinions, and reassures you against ridicule and vituperative remarks. See Appendix A for a list of additional books, videos and websites.

My people are destroyed through lack of knowledge. Hosea 4:6

Don't be discouraged by difficulties you encounter starting on a health conscious vegetarian diet. Your taste buds may have been conditioned to a high fat, high salt, high sugar diet. It takes only a short time to recondition them to a healthier eating regime. You'll be enjoying your new diet in 3 to 6 weeks. Give it a chance! Your reward will be excellent health and energy.

Finally, find other vegetarians. Maybe join a vegetarian/vegan society. If you are a new vegetarian, other vegetarians will be more than willing to give you support, encouragement and advice. You can exchange recipes, discuss vegetarian issues and have vegetarian dinner parties.

Is it difficult to give up meat?

Vegetarians are not supermen or women, and do not possess any greater willpower than meat-eaters. It is thought by many contemplating making the move to a vegetarian diet that they simply could not give up meat, and find it difficult to comprehend the "sacrifice" vegetarians have made. Without doubt, the benefits of a vegetarian diet far outweigh the giving up of animal products!

The good news, however, is that it is easier than you might think. All it takes is a conscience decision and a short period of only a few weeks to break longstanding habits. If you had asked me prior to November 2000 that I would become a vegan, and that I would write this book, no doubt you would have been heartily laughed at. Once that determined decision is made, it is not difficult at all. And that is good news!

Where do I buy vegetarian food?

Exactly the same place you currently buy food. Of course, much of what is available in supermarkets are animal foods or animal based foods. These no longer have any sway with you. On the positive side, due to the increasing popularity of vegetarianism, vegetarian foods are now more widely available. And don't forget your local greengrocer who works so hard to bring you the freshest available produce.

Will I get all the vital nutrients and minerals?

Certainly. A well balanced, low-fat vegetarian diet based on the New Four Food Groups: Fruits, Vegetables, Legumes and Whole Grains. These provide sufficient vitamins (remember to find a source of Vitamin B_{12}, such as fortified soy milk or supplementation), minerals, fiber and other essential phytonutrients. As long as you are eating a balanced vegetarian diet you will not need to buy expensive vitamin supplements.

Remember Daniel's successful vegetarian result...

And at the end of ten days their countenance appeared better and fatter in flesh than all the young me who ate the portion of the king's delicacies. Daniel 1:15

It is a myth that vegetarians are pale, anemic and scraggy. In fact, the contrary is true. Because of the dramatically reduced toxicity in the body, vegetarians exhibit a skin tone that radiates good health. As for calcium, vegetarian diets contain adequate amounts from leafy green vegetables, tofu, beans and nuts.

Isn't vegetarian food boring?

Be assured that vegetarians do not lead miserable lives eating lettuce and carrots every day. With hundreds of available fruits, vegetables, nuts, seeds and grains, a wonderful array of delicious and nutritious meals are available for you to try. There are vegetarian societies, books, magazines and the internet where you can find delicious and nutritious recipes, cooking tips and tricks. Indeed, because vegetarians are generally far more aware of nutrition and its relationship to good health, they tend to be more passionate about what they do in terms of food preparation.

Is vegetarian cooking difficult?

Like any cuisine, vegetarian cooking can range from very simple to the more extravagant. Generally, however, vegetarian cooking is simpler and easier and usually does not take as long. Vegetarian soups are very easy to make, and what could be easier than eating some fruit for breakfast?

Will I be ridiculed by my friends and work colleagues?

You might be, but so what? Whose health are you concerned about, yours or theirs? Be true to your convictions, and they will respect you for it, particularly when they see how much your health has improved and how much weight you have lost. This is where reading and learning as much about vegetarianism comes in useful!

What about when I travel?

Yes, this can be a problem sometimes, particularly when arriving late at night and nothing else open but fast food restaurants. When traveling, pack vegetarian snacks such as soups, fresh fruit and vegetables, dried fruit and nuts, crackers, etc. Fill a cooler with sandwiches and containers of juice or soy milk.

Can I raise children on a vegetarian diet?

Certainly. All issues relating to adults also apply to

children. In fact, the shocking truth is that many of the degenerative diseases we experience in later life actually begin when we are children, where poor eating habits are picked up from parents and family.

Pediatrician, Dr Alan Attwood, MD, was so concerned about the incidence of death by coronary heart disease and cancer that he dedicated himself to the prevention of these diseases through nutrition, particularly in children. Dr Attwood presents a number of myths regarding raising children on a low-fat vegetarian diet.[7]

Myth 1: *Controlling Cholesterol Can Wait.* Some 4 out of 10 children have high cholesterol levels. These high cholesterol levels result in fatty deposits in the heart arteries, resulting in heart attacks later on in adult life. Cholesterol levels should be controlled in children so that the probability of having raised levels later in life is minimized.

Myth 2: *Controlling Obesity Can Wait.* Childhood obesity is increasing, with some 1 in 4 being overweight. Obese children rarely 'grow out of it' and continue to stack on the weight into adulthood. The overweight child, whose parents are waiting for him to become slim when he grows older, is probably a victim of too much fatty food and lack of exercise.

Myth 3: *The 'Fat Taste' Is Natural and Inborn.* There are no fat taste buds, only sweet, salty, sour and bitter. Fat is 'tasted' through a combination of senses, such as smell and the food's sensation of smoothness on the tongue and throat. Children are not born with a taste for fat. It is established by repeated exposure with pleasant experience and social events. To emphasize this, what is served at a child's birthday party - cakes or broccoli? Fat in a child's diet should be eliminated as much as possible.

Myth 4: *Small Reductions in Fat Will Do.* Moderate reductions in fat do not effectively eliminate a child's 'taste' for fat, nor will this significantly reduce the risk of coronary heart disease later in life. Trimming fat from meat or removing the skin from chicken is not enough. No more than 10% of calories should be obtained from fat. This is not possible when children eat meat, dairy products and eggs. Only a low-fat vegan diet can achieve this low level of fat consumption.

Myth 5: *Childrens' Diets are Getting Better.* Look no further to the proliferation of fast food outlets to see the changing demands for more and more fatty foods. There is no doubt that children's diets are getting worse, not better, as the fat rampage continues.

Myth 6: *Meat is Needed for Protein and Iron.* In western countries, meat has attained an unprecedented status among consumers, but meat is not necessary to ensure a supply of protein and iron. The daily requirement for protein is actually quite low - some 40g per day for children and 60g per day for adults, while iron requirements are 8mg and 12mg respectively. These levels are easily obtained by eating a varied vegetarian diet containing leafy greens, legumes and grains. There is no need for animal sources of protein and iron.

Myth 7: *Milk is Needed for Calcium.* One of the biggest scare campaigns to come from the dairy industry is that dairy is necessary for strong bones. Yet milk is such an unnecessary source of calcium and spoils a perfect diet. When dairy products are removed from children's diets, many allergies are reduced. Dairy milk has also been linked to Type I diabetes in children (for more information regarding dairy products, see Osteoporosis in the previous chapter).

My daughter, Katrina, at one time consistently suffered from earaches and bronchitis. Many a night you could hear her coughing and crying with the pain. We took her to the doctor many times, who promptly prescribed antibiotics, but the conditions would always recur. The doctor even wanted her to undergo an operation to enlarge her sinuses and put tubes in her ears. To my wife's credit, she felt the Lord say no to this, to which I am eternally grateful. The good news is that, when we stopped feeding Katrina milk and dairy products, there was no more recurrence of earaches and bronchitis, truly an amazing turnaround and answer to prayer!

There is no age barrier to the benefits of giving up dairy consumption. Dr Benjamin Spock, MD, famous for his book, Dr Spock's Baby and Child Care, which has been a key reference to parents for 60 years with over 50 million copies in print, relates a similar experience of giving up dairy products at the ripe old age of 88...[8]

> *Seven years ago, I made major changes in my own diet. At 88 years of age, I began a nondairy, low-fat diet. Within two weeks, my chronic bronchitis went away after years of unsuccessful antibiotic treatments. I know many people who have used nutritional changes to deal successfully with very serious conditions, including heart disease and cancer. [Dr Benjamin Spock]*

Myth 8: *Low Fat Diets Lack Vitamins and Minerals.* A child's diet, rich in varied plant foods from the New Four Food Groups, is not deficient in vitamins and minerals.

Myth 9: *Low Fat Diets Mean Limited Choices.* A diet rich in fruits, vegetables, legumes and grains is more satisfying than one high in fat and animal foods. With a little sense of adventure, wonderful meals can be prepared giving a huge amount of variety and satisfaction.

Myth 10: *Low Fat Diets Retard Growth.* There is no doubt that children consuming a low-fat plant based diet will grow to their full potential adult height. However, an animal based diet may, in fact, retard growth. For example, it is known that children in meat eating societies reach menarche (first menstruation) at an earlier age, which is then accompanied by a slow down in growth.

Hormones added to animal feed are a major factor in the current trend to earlier menarche...[9]

> *Cow's milk has a high fat content, high levels of biologically available hormones and growth factors, and other chemical contaminants from highly medicated cows fed environmental trash (chicken feces and diseased carcasses, for instance). These are all linked to early puberty and proliferation of cancer cells in human reproductive organs. [Dr Linda Palmer]*

One study specifically found that girls with early menarche had deleterious changes in insulin, glucose, blood pressure and body fat levels than girls with average or late menarche. It also found that early menarche adversely affected cardiovascular disease risk factor, elevated blood pressure and glucose intolerance.[10]

Raw Foods

The processed food industry is big business, as any casual observation at the supermarket will attest to. Row upon row of supermarket shelves show all kinds of boxes and packages full of foods that do not look anything like what can be found growing from the ground or on a tree. Cutting down on processed foods to a minimum is a key measure in combating the increased incidence of chronic disease and obesity. The convenience of processed foods simply does not justify the poor nutrition they provide.

Wanton spending on processed foods only encourages the growth of this market. Furthermore, most processed foods are actually quite expensive, and when compared on a nutrition-per-dollar basis, they mostly compare very unfavorably with fresh fruits and vegetables.

Often described as dead food, processed foods usually contain a high proportion of fat, sugar, flavor enhancers and other unhealthy chemical additives (food additives are discussed in greater detail later in this chapter). The refinement and manufacturing processes takes a lot of the nutrients out of the food leaving a bulky mass that contains little or no beneficial nutrition. Mostly, processed foods become nothing more than unhealthy filling for the stomach.

On the other hand, raw plant foods contain the highest levels of enzymes, which act as catalysts for thousands of important chemical reactions in the body. When food is cooked, even over a relatively cool temperature (in terms of cooking temperatures), most of the enzymes in the food are destroyed. Enzymes are often referred to as the life-force or energy of the food.

Dr Norman Walker, DSc, a pioneer in modern health science, explains the importance of live enzymes to our health...[11]

> *The basic key to the efficacy of nourishing your body is the life which is present in your food and of those intangible elements, known as enzymes. In other words, the element which enables the body to be nourished and live, that element which is hidden within the seeds of plants and in the sprouting and growth of plants is a life principle known as enzymes. [Dr Norman Walker]*

There is no specific recommendation as to what percentage of the diet should be from raw foods, although the higher the percentage, the greater the health benefits. Some people say that we should eat a 100% raw food diet, however, this means you would not be able to eat many beneficial foods that need to be cooked, such as beans, breads and many vegetables. Some vegetables are too bitter to be eaten raw, such as parsnips, turnips and potatoes, but when cooked, are delicious and nutritious.

It is quite easy to eat 60 to 70%, even 80%, of our diet as raw food, as the following sample day indicates...

Meal	**Sample Menu**
Breakfast	Fresh vegetable juice (see Juicing in the next chapter) and some fruit.
Lunch	Salad sandwich (no butter!) with wholemeal bread (why not two salad sandwiches?).
Snack	Piece of fruit or a vegetable (such as a carrot).
Dinner	Baked potatoes, steamed rice, lentils and a side salad.
Evening	Piece of fruit, raw nuts.

It should be noted that not all processed foods are deleterious to health. After all, who would argue that freshly baked wholemeal bread, when eaten in moderation, is not good for us? Thus, it is necessary to be judicious in our choices of processed foods. It all depends on how highly processed the food is and what ingredients it contains.

Of course, the key is to be flexible, without making difficult rules for yourself that you can't keep! Some days less raw food will be eaten, other days, more.

Animal Foods

In today's modern world, it is easy to forget that the flesh we buy was once part of living, breathing animals. With animals being killed and their meat being butchered in abattoirs located in places far away, there is a sense of complacency about the origin of our meat. Like Sergeant Shultz of Hogan's Heroes fame, it's almost a case of "I know nussing"!

In a lifetime, a human can eat thousands of animals such as chickens, cows, pigs and fish. That's a lot of protein, fat, cholesterol and concentrations of antibiotics, herbicides and pesticides for the body to deal with.

Humans are often described as omnivores, however, this is only based on the observation that humans eat meat as well as plants. However, comparisons between the anatomies of herbivores and carnivores show striking differences, and indeed, humans have all the features of herbivores. The following table comprehensively shows these comparisons...[12]

Facial Muscles

Carnivore:	Reduced to allow wide mouth gape
Herbivore:	Well developed
Human:	Same as herbivore

Jaw Type

Carnivore:	Angle not expanded
Herbivore:	Expanded angle
Human:	Same as herbivore

Jaw Joint Location

Carnivore:	On same plane as molar teeth
Herbivore:	Above the plane of molars
Human:	Same as herbivore

Jaw Motion

Carnivore: Shearing, minimal side to side motion
Herbivore: No shearing, side-to-side, front-to-back
Human: Same as herbivore

Major Jaw Muscles

Carnivore: Temporalis
Herbivore: Masseter and pterygoids
Human: Same as herbivore

Mouth Opening vs Head Size

Carnivore: Large
Herbivore: Small
Human: Same as herbivore

Teeth (incisors)

Carnivore: Short and pointed
Herbivore: Short, flattened and spade shaped
Human: Same as herbivore

Teeth (canines)

Carnivore: Long, sharp and curved
Herbivore: Dull and short
Human: Short and blunted

Teeth (molars)

Carnivore: Sharp, jagged and blade shaped
Herbivore: Flattened with cusps
Human: Flattened with nodular cusps

Chewing
Carnivore: None, swallows food whole
Herbivore: Extensive chewing necessary
Human: Same as herbivore

Saliva
Carnivore: No digestive enzymes
Herbivore: Carbohydrate digestive enzymes
Human: Same as herbivore

Stomach Acidity
Carnivore: Less than pH 1
Herbivore: pH 4 to 5
Human: Same as herbivore

Stomach Capacity
Carnivore: 60 to 70% of total volume of digestive tract
Herbivore: Less than 30% of total volume of digestive tract
Human: Same as herbivore

Length of Small Intestines
Carnivore: 3 to 6 times body length
Herbivore: 10 to more than 12 times body length
Human: 10 to 11 times body length

Colon
Carnivore: Simple, short and smooth
Herbivore: Long, complex; may be sacculated
Human: Long, sacculated

Liver
    Carnivore: Can detoxify vitamin A
    Herbivore: Cannot detoxify vitamin A
    Human: Same as herbivore

Kidney
    Carnivore: Concentrated urine
    Herbivore: Moderately concentrated urine
    Human: Same as herbivore

Nails
    Carnivore: Sharp claws
    Herbivore: Flattened nails or blunt hooves
    Human: Flattened nails

In every physiological characteristic, man is a vegetarian, as originally created by God. We are not made up to kill animals, and without guns, traps, tools and fire, we would find it very difficult, if not impossible, to hunt animals for food. We do not possess the claws or strong jaws and teeth that can rip through the hide of an animal and tear its flesh. Could a man pounce on an animal in the wild, tear its limbs apart while the animal is still alive, suck the living blood from it, then dive his face into its carcass to rip out flesh, tissues and organs?

Of course not! Instead, the human hand is very adept at simply picking fruit from trees and vines. Our natural instincts are non-carnivorous, and the thought of killing, skinning and boning animals is repugnant to most people. We simply just allow others to do it. Would you be able to eat pork if you had to kill and bone the pig yourself?

Have you ever had that tired feeling after a huge meal? You know the drill - you go to your in-law's for Christmas dinner and they bring out so much food that you have difficulty eating it all. There is meat loaf, ham, chicken, turkey, cheese and salads containing lots of meat portions. Afterwards, you feel tired and just want to have an hour's nap.

Do not join those who drink too much wine or gorge themselves on meat, for drunkards and gluttons become poor, and drowsiness clothes them in rags. Proverbs 23:20-21

The drowsiness comes about for two reasons: (1) tremendous amounts of energy are required to digest animal protein and fat, and (2) sludging and slowing of the blood deprives the body of energy and oxygen. The digestion of proteins is a much "dirtier" process than digesting the carbohydrates of plants, with ammonia being the chief waste product. It is a cumbersome way of extracting energy from food.

Apart from not being part of God's original diet, animal foods are not particularly helpful because they have no fiber, no complex starchy carbohydrates and none of the primary antioxidant vitamins such as vitamin C, E and beta-carotene, and no vitamin K.[13] Even the leanest portion of meat is marbled with high levels of fat and cholesterol. For this reason, meat does not offer much protection against heart disease, cancer and diabetes, as do fruits and vegetables. For example, meat does contain vitamin A but not in its precursor beta-carotene form, and therefore lacks the immune-boosting effects of this antioxidant.

Animal foods contain high levels of saturated fat. Apart from the difficulty in digesting and metabolizing these fats, once inside the bloodstream, saturated fat is converted to very-low-density lipoproteins (VLDL), which are then transformed into low-density lipoproteins (LDL), the so-called "bad cholesterol." Cholesterol comes only from animal foods, but does not exist at all in plant foods. Even olive oil, which is 100% oil (mostly unsaturated), contains no cholesterol.

Low density lipoproteins contribute to the formation of thick, hard deposits on arterial walls called plaques. These plaques harden the arterial walls and narrow the artery itself, a condition known as atherosclerosis. By way of comparison, "good cholesterol," or high-density lipoproteins (HDL), have a tendency to carry cholesterol away from arteries back into the liver, where they are passed out from the body via the large intestine.

Moreover, digestive remains of animal products tend to stick to the inner linings of the intestines and putrefy due to lack of fiber. This makes it more difficult for spent cholesterol to pass through the intestinal wall for elimination, the depleted fiber levels reducing its absorption.

Deceptive Foods

In today's modern Western society, we look on God's original plant based vegetarian diet as a quirk by health-freaks, but have failed to understand the significance of it. Our western diet is too high in fats, oils, sugars, salts and processed foods, all of which were never intended for us to eat in the quantities we consume today.

Many of today's foods are deceptive and have little or no nutritional value. In fact, many are quite harmful. These so-called foods are manufactured, processed, artificially colored, artificially flavored, chemically treated, re-constituted, genetically modified, pasteurized, homogenized, powdered, dehydrated, irradiated, etc. Is this what God intended when He created the Garden of Eden?

Scripture warns against excessive eating, or gluttony, as well as warning us against eating these delicacies and deceptive foods.

When you sit down to eat with a ruler, consider carefully what is before you. And

put a knife to your throat if you are a man given to appetite. Do not desire his delicacies, for they are deceptive food. Proverbs 23:1-3

The appetite of King Henry VIII is legendary. Living in a time of profound changes in European cuisine, explorers would return with strange new foods from the Far East and the New World. These foods were skillfully crafted by Henry's kitchen staff to produce outrageous dishes, including peacock pies, alcoholic beverages spiked with gold, and magnificently sculptured sugar desserts. King Henry, once a healthy and athletic young man, grew to an enormous 54 inches around the waist![14]

We need to return to the Garden for our food!

History of Deceptive Foods

When examining the history of deceptive foods, it is interesting to note that many of their origins and developments are similar. They were mostly unknown to the Christian world, generally unheard of even just a few centuries ago, and were usually associated with pagan worship or regarded for medicinal purposes. Some deceptive foods were not well accepted at first, but with a little experimentation, formulas were developed causing their popularity to spread quickly.

Many deceptive foods were in the enclave of the rich, who spurned natural foods for their deceptive foods. The poor, often envious of the privileged classes, coveted these foods for themselves. Some were catalysts for political intrigue and the pursuit of wealth and power, even to the point of triggering wars and rebellion.

Finally, many deceptive foods were made available to all levels of society as the industrial revolution and mass-manufacturing techniques began to bring prices down. Working class citizens now had access to deceptive foods only the wealthy could previously afford. These foods began to be consumed in enormous quantities far in excess of what the body can adequately tolerate.

Chewing Gum

Chewing gum has its origins from a number of different sources. The ancient Greeks chewed a resin from the mastic tree called mastiche (mas-tee-ka), the ancient Mayans chewed chicle which is the sap from the sapodilla tree, and North American Indians chewed sap from spruce trees, passing on the practice to early American settlers.

In 1845, Thomas Adams began experimenting with spruce gum as a rubber substitute. These experiments where not successful, and in frustration, Adams inserted some chicle into his mouth and struck up the idea to flavor it. Shortly thereafter, Adams opened the world's first chewing gum factory called State of Maine Pure Spruce Gum. However, by 1850, flavored paraffin gums became more popular than spruce gums. By 1869, the first chewing gum was patented.

In 1888, a chewing gum called Tutti Frutti was the first to be sold in vending machines located in New York City's subway stations. By 1906, the first bubble gum was developed. In 1928, while experimenting with new gum recipes, Walter Diemer invented the successful pink colored bubble gum. It was pink because that was the only shade of food coloring that he had available at the time.

Chewing gum is not part of God's original diet.

Chocolate

During the conquest of Mexico, Cortez found that Aztec Indians used cocoa beans to make a drink known as chocolatl meaning "warm liquid." This concoction was sacred and associated with fertility and wisdom.

In 1519, Emperor Montezuma served chocolatl to his

Spanish guests as a food for the gods. However, the drink was very bitter and to make it more agreeable, sugar was added to sweeten it. Other innovations included adding cinnamon and vanilla, as well as serving the drink hot.

The new drink became very popular, especially amongst the Spanish aristocracy, and so the cocoa industry was born. Chocolatl then became very popular throughout Europe as a health tonic.

The invention of the steam engine allowed chocolatl to be mass-produced using mechanized cocoa-grinding processes, greatly reducing its price. The cocoa press, invented in 1828, helped to improve the quality of the beverage by extruding out the cocoa butter (cocoa bean fat). In 1847, an English company introduced solid eating chocolate, and in 1876, milk was added to form what we know today as milk chocolate.

Chocolate is not part of God's original diet.

Coffee

The effects of coffee were first noticed by a humble shepherd in Kaffa, Ethiopia (hence the origin of the word coffee), when his sheep would become hyperactive after eating a certain red berry. By about 1000 AD, tribes in Ethiopia noticed they got an energy boost by grinding and eating the red berry. It was about this time that Arab traders took coffee back to their homelands and cultivated it in the first coffee plantations. They boiled the beans to create a drink that helped them stay awake.

In the early 1500's, coffee made its way to Constantinople by Ottoman Turks. Here coffee beans were roasted for the first time over open fires, then crushed and boiled in water, creating a crude version of the modern day cup of coffee. The first coffee house was opened in Turkey in 1554. By 1600, coffee entered Europe via the port of Venice by Italian traders and Pope Clement VIII "baptizes" it despite Christian opposition to the "devil's drink." In the next few decades, coffee houses began spreading all over Europe, with coffee becoming a popular breakfast beverage. The famous insurance company Lloyd's of London had its origins in Edward Lloyd's coffee house frequented by merchants and maritime insurance representatives.

In 1675, the habit of filtering ground coffee and adding milk was established, with sugar being added a little while later.

In the United States the Continental Congress declared coffee a national drink in protest against excessive taxes on tea levied by the British government. The Boston Tea Party of 1773 declared drinking coffee a patriotic duty in America.

In the late 1800's and early 1900's, mass-manufacture of instant and freeze-dried coffee began to replace local roasting shops and coffee mills. Coffee machines such as the Expresso and filter drip coffee makers appeared.

Today, coffee is the world's most popular beverage, and the coffee industry has become a global giant ranking second only to oil in terms of world trade value.

Coffee is not part of God's original diet.

Confectionery

The word candy comes from the Arab word qandi, meaning a lump of sugar cane. Today, candy covers a range of sweets with sugar as the main ingredient.

Honey was an important ingredient in ancient candy, with the Egyptians, Arabs and Chinese making confections of fruits and nuts candied in honey.

During the Middle Ages, only the wealthy could afford candy because of the high cost of sugar, however, the discovery of sugar beet juice as a sweetener and the onset of the industrial revolution allowed the candy industry to flourish when popular penny candies such as peppermints and lemon drops were sold.

Today, there are thousands of recipes for confectionaries such as candy, chocolate bars, toffees, lollies, lollypops, popsicles, desserts, nougats, etc. For many people, confectionery forms a significant part of their diet.

Confectionery is not part of God's original diet.

Hamburgers

In the early 1200's, the Mongol horsemen led by Genghis Khan ate raw ground mutton or lamb while riding on their horses. Khan's grandson, Kubilai Khan, brought this unique dietary ground meat with him when he invaded Moscow. The Russians adopted this meat into their own cuisine by adding chopped onions and eggs, calling it steak tartare (tartare is the Russian word for Mongols).

When German ships from Hamburg began calling on Russian ports during the 1600's, Russian steak tartare was brought back to Germany. By the 18th century, the term Hamburg Steak came into popular usage. German immigrants to America brought with them recipes for Hamburg Steak consisting of minced low-grade beef cooked into patties with chopped onions, breadcrumbs and spices. These patties were quickly cooked on a grill and eaten between two pieces of bread. American restaurants soon began offering hamburger steak as an affordable meal.

Just who is responsible for the hamburger in a bun as we know it today is the subject of some debate, with many different stories and claims. What is known, however, is that the hamburger created a sensation in the 1904 St Louis World Fair. By 1931, a cartoon character known as Wimpy Wimpy joined the Popeye comic strip. Known for his insatiable consumption of hamburgers, Wimpy Wimpy popularized the hamburger in the United States, even spawning a chain of hamburger restaurants called Wimpy's.

Today, hamburgers are sold by the millions around the world every day. They are not part of God's original diet.

Ice Cream

The first frozen ice dessert was a mixture of snow, fruit pulp and honey mixed together for Emperor Nero of Rome. Marco Polo was also said to have brought with him from the Far East recipes of water ices used in Asia for thousands of years.

In the 15th century, Catherine de Medici brought the sorbet concept to France. Later in France, it was discovered that custard made a delectable dessert when frozen. This was followed shortly thereafter by the invention of a machine that made a superior frozen custard.

Upon hearing about the new dessert, Dolly Madison, the wife of US President James Madison, made ice cream a feature of dinners at the White House.

In 1851 the first ice-cream factory was built in Baltimore, USA, and so, commercial ice-cream's time had come. In 1903, the ice-cream cone was developed by Italo Marchiony when he reduced his overheads by baking edible waffle cups to serve his ice-cream, rather than customers running off with his serving glasses.

At the turn of the 19th century, ice-cream was accidentally dropped into soda water, and so the ice-cream soda was born. Fearing that the national craze for ice-cream soda made young people too amorous while courting over a drink, the sale of ice-cream soda was banned on Sundays. However, an enterprising druggist concocted a legal alternative containing ice cream and syrup, calling it sundae.

For over a century now, manufacturers of ice-cream have invented many ingenious ways of selling their product, from ice-cream cones to buckets, with literally hundreds of different and sometimes exotic flavors.

Ice cream is not part of God's original diet.

Lemonade

It appears that lemonade had its origins in the tenth

century Egyptian peasantry. Although use of the lemon itself originated much earlier, medieval Jewish communities in Cairo bottled lemon juice and sugar in a beverage known as qatarmizat, which was consumed locally and exported.

The first marketed lemonades appeared in the 17th century and were made from water and lemon juice sweetened with honey or sugar. In 1676, the Compagnie de Limonadiers of Paris was granted a monopoly for the sale of lemonade soft drinks. Vendors carried tanks of lemonade on their backs and dispensed cups of the beverage to thirsty Parisians

Bathing in natural mineral springs has long been considered a healthy thing to do, and mineral water itself is said to have curative powers. However, scientists soon discovered that carbon dioxide created the bubbles in mineral water. This led the Swedish chemist Torbern Bergman in 1770 to invent an apparatus for artificially ingesting carbon dioxide into water thereby producing imitation mineral water in large quantities. This led to a patent in the US for the means of mass-manufacture of imitation mineral waters and soda waters.

As the practice of drinking natural or artificial mineral water was considered healthy, chemists soon started adding other ingredients such as sarsaparilla and fruit extracts. Early drug stores sold their drink from soda fountains, and in order to satisfy customers' demands to take home the drink with them, the drink bottling industry was born. In the 1920's the Hom-Pak, the precursor to the six-pack, was available.

Lemonade is not part of God's original diet.

Margarine

Margarine was first manufactured by a French food research chemist in response to Napoleon's request for an economical, longer-lasting alternative to butter. From these beginnings, commercial production of margarine began in the 1870's and its popularity grew.

Margarine gets its name from the Greek word margarites, meaning pearl, because of the shiny pearly drops of oil extruded from the purified animal fat from which margarine was originally made.

In the following decades, the proportion of animal fat in margarine decreased and vegetable oils increased. Further processing refinements, particularly the ability to convert vegetable oils to solid fats (known as trans-fats) by the process of 'hydrogenation' (ie, saturation of the oil with hydrogen), enabled margarine to be made entirely from vegetable sources. The most common oils used today for margarine manufacture are rapeseed, sunflower, soy and palm.

The process of manufacturing margarine is very complex...[15]

Oil Extraction and Refinement: Seeds are washed, crushed and heated and the oil removed in a solvent extraction process. The crude oil is neutralized to remove free fatty acids that would otherwise react with oxygen and give the oil a rancid taste. Colors and impurities are removed by passing a special absorbent earth through the oil. A process known as rearrangement, where different oils are combined and blended, is used to produce a fat with different melting characteristics. Steam is also passed through the heated oil to remove unwanted smells and tastes from the oil.

Product Manufacture: A fractionation and separation process is used to cool the oil so that harder oils crystallize and separate out from the softer part. Rearrangement and esterification use a combination of high temperatures and pressure to concentrate the oil molecules in order to make them harder. Hydrogenation is also used to alter the original molecular structure of the oil by passing hydrogen gas through at high temperature and pressure. Catalysts are used to speed up these processes. Variations in these processes are employed to give different textures and properties of the hardened oil, which is blended and agitated with other ingredients such as vitamins, colors, flavors, emulsifiers, whey, brine, milk proteins and starches. Finally, the product is chilled and kneaded to form margarine as we know it.

Margarine is today no doubt a prime example of a deceptive manufactured food, and is not part of God's original diet.

Refrigeration
Refrigeration is mentioned here due to its profound affect in the ability to store and preserve foods for much longer. Meats that went off in only a few hours or days could now be frozen and stored for many months, allowing greater quantities of meat to be kept in the home. Dairy products previously unable to be kept for very long were now able to be stored in greater quantities.

The earliest forms of refrigeration used by the Hebrews, Greeks and Romans required the placement of large amounts of snow into storage pits with insulating coverings. Cooling drinks such as iced liquors and frozen juices came into vogue in Europe's warmer southern climates, and by 1600, long-necked bottles were immersed in water in which saltpeter was dissolved.

Prior to 1830, food preservation consisted of salting, smoking, pickling or drying. However, rapid growth of cities and general economic improvement of the population increased the demand for fresh produce, which needed to be transported from even greater distances. Refrigerated railway carriages came into widespread use.

Early refrigeration was recognized by the brewing industry, allowing breweries to make more uniform products all year round. A short time after that, the meat-packing industry adopted refrigeration in a big way.

Soon, almost every industry used refrigeration from

storage of raw ingredients to distribution of the final product. Refrigeration provided a boon to florists, mortuaries, confectioners, chocolate and ice-cream makers, dairy producers, meat packers, drug companies, hospitals, and many others.

Over the last 150 years, great advances in refrigeration have been made, allowing the cooling and freezing of food products and medicines over longer periods of time. Today, the humble household refrigerator is taken for granted, however, it dramatically changed the way people ate and affected society in a profound manner. By the 1920's the household refrigerator was an essential appliance in the kitchen.

Salt

The ancient Hebrews used salt as part of their sacrifice to the Lord (Leviticus 2:13), of which they had an inexhaustible and ready supply of it on the southern shores of the Dead Sea. It was considered a symbol of purity and incorruptibility. Offering bread and salt to visitors was an important etiquette in many cultures, and made for unbreakable friendship and bonding. To Christians, salt seasoning is compared with temperance of speech…

> **Let your speech always be with grace, seasoned with salt, that you may know how you ought to answer each one. Colossians 4:6**

So valuable was salt to earlier civilizations that it has served as currency, and has even provided the basis for conflicts and wars. It was important politically, economically and socially for thousands of years. So important was salt that Jesus equated it with the effectiveness of God's people…

> **You are the salt of the earth, but if the salt**

loses its flavor, how shall it be seasoned? It is then good for nothing but to be thrown out and trampled underfoot by men. Matthew 5:13

The expression "not worth his salt" comes from the exchange of slaves for salt in ancient Greece. Special salt rations, known as salarium argentums (the precursor of the word salary) were given to early Roman soldiers. Salt was an important commodity carried to newly discovered countries by explorers. Mahatma Ghandi led thousands of Indians on an exhausting 240-mile march to the sea to make their own salt in protest over salt taxes. Although Ghandi was jailed, the march began a series of events that led to the ending of British rule over India.

Salt has over 14,000 known uses. The greatest single use of salt by far is for the production of chemicals. The second highest use of salt is water conditioning, and the third road de-icing. Only about 6% of salt is used as a food additive and flavoring. [16]

Sodium is an essential mineral, however, to be usable in the body, it must be ingested from naturally occurring organic sodium compounds. Ingesting additional salt from purified sodium chloride (table salt) is neither necessary nor beneficial to health. Excessive salt intake has a direct affect on blood pressure, and causes the retention of water in order to keep the salt in solution, leading to swelling of ankles and joints as well as weight gain. Too much salt also increases the risk of osteoporosis, heart disease, stroke and other health issues.[17]

Paul C. Bragg, ND, pioneer of the health movement in America, says this about salt...[18]

Salt cannot be digested, assimilated or utilized by the body. Salt has no nutritional value! Salt has no vitamins, no organic minerals and no nutrients of any kind!

Instead, it is harmful and causes trouble in the kidneys, bladder, heart, arteries, veins and blood vessels. Salt is the main cause of waterlogged tissues that cause swelling and edema (dropsy). [Dr Paul Bragg, ND]

It is estimated that each western citizen consumes up to 16 tons in a lifetime.[19] In fact, only a small proportion of salt is added to food and cooking in the home, the majority is added to processed foods, the so-called "hidden salt."

Job asked the rhetorical question: "Can flavorless food be eaten without salt?" (Job 6:6). The answer is, Yes! There are many wonderful herbs and spices that can be added to foods to enhance their flavor.

Smoking

While not a food, of course, smoking is such an influence on ill health, that its inclusion here is warranted.

Tobacco was first grown in the Americas, and it was about 1,000 BC when native Indians began to use the leaves for smoking and chewing. How it was discovered that tobacco could be smoked or chewed is not certain, however, it is believed that tobacco leaves were used to care for wounds and relieve pain. Most likely, tobacco smoking formed part of the pagan rites of the Indians. When the Mayan civilizations dispersed, the scattered tribes brought their tobacco with them.

In 1492, Christopher Columbus was the first outsider to come in contact with tobacco. Later that year, Rodrigo de Jerez landed on Cuba and witnessed locals wrapping tobacco leaves in palm or maize, lighting one end and inhaling smoke. Jerez was the first smoker in Europe, and in 1493, shocked the Spanish who saw smoke coming out of his mouth and nose. They thought he was demon-possessed and imprisoned him for seven years. By the time of his release, however, smoking had become acceptable in Spain.

Soon, tobacco was cultivated by Europeans in the Caribbean, and its popularity increased in most European nations. In 1560, Jean Nicot de Villemain advanced smoking as a cure-all. It was Villemain who gave his name to the word nicotine.

Smoking was not universally accepted, though. In 1604, King James I published his "Counterblaste to Tobacco," labeling it as "an invention from Satan" and banned tobacco from London's public bars. However, he was later forced to nationalize the uncontrollable tobacco trade and raised tobacco taxes to unprecedented levels as a repressive measure. It is speculated that James I had Sir Walter Raleigh executed because he held Raleigh responsible for introducing tobacco into England.

Pope Clement VIII threatened anyone caught smoking in a holy place with excommunication. Michael Feodorovich, the first Csar of Russia, declared the use of tobacco a deadly sin and forbade possession for any purpose. In Turkey, Persia and India, the death penalty applied.

Despite these measures, through the 16th and 17th centuries, tobacco and pipe smoking became almost universal. Cuban style cigars also became very popular in Spain but not so in the rest of Europe until the 19th century. In 1832, the first paper rolled cigarettes were made, it is believed, by Egyptian soldiers fighting the Turkish/Egyptian war. From this, commercialization of tobacco, particularly that of cigarettes, increased in the 18th century.

The first medical warnings against the effects of smoking were raised by the medical journal The Lancet in 1858. By the late 1800's prohibition existed in many US states as well as calls to label tobacco products with the word "poison." In 1950, evidence of a link between smoking and lung cancer was established, and by the 1980's, many western countries banned the advertising of cigarettes and tobacco products.

This was followed by smoking bans in restaurants, public transport, work places, and public buildings.

Sugar

It is understood that sugar dates back several thousand years to New Guinea and then spread along South East Asia to India. It was about 500 BC when the process of pressing out the juice of the cane and boiling it into crystals was developed in India.

Sugar cultivation was not introduced into Europe until the Middle Ages, when the Crusaders in the 11th century returned home talking about sugar and how pleasant it was. In 1319, sugar was available in London at "two schillings a pound," which probably equates to about $100 per kg at today's prices.

Christopher Columbus took sugar cane plants to the Caribbean, where the climate was advantageous to its growth. By this time, governments recognized the vast profits to be made from sugar production, and taxed it highly. This situation remained in force until about 1815, when sugar taxes were abolished to bring the price of sugar within the means of the ordinary citizen.

Sugar, in its refined state, is not part of God's original diet.

Tea

Tea has its origins in ancient China some 5,000 years ago. It was not until 800AD, however, that Lu Yu, raised and trained by Buddhist monks, codified the cultivation and preparation of tea.

A Buddhist priest brought tea into Japan from China in order to enhance religious meditation. Tea drinking spread rapidly to all levels of society throughout Japan. Teahouses became very popular, with even the Geisha specializing in the presentation of the tea ceremony.

Tea finally arrived in Europe during the reign of Elizabeth I, when it became very fashionable. But due to its high cost, it remained within the domain of the wealthy. Slowly, as the amount of tea imported increased, the price began to fall making it available to all levels of society.

The ubiquitous tea tax became the focus of America's desire for freedom over their oppressive English overlords. As the colonists rebelled and openly purchased contraband tea, the largest tea company in the world, the British East India Company, saw profits fall resulting in serious financial difficulty. The company was given permission to sell directly to the colonists, however, the colonists refused to drink it, turning to coffee instead. By 1773, the situation had deteriorated so badly that 60 men of Boston, dressed as Mohawk Indians, dumped thousands of pounds worth of tea into the ocean (an event known as the Boston Tea Party), thus beginning the violent dispute between America and England culminating in the War of Independence.

In more modern times, variations in tea drinking came into vogue. Iced tea made its debut in 1904 when a tea plantation owner put ice in his tea samples at the World Fair in St Louis. Four years later, a tea merchant developed bagged tea as restaurant samples, but found that the restaurants were brewing the tea in the bags to avoid a mess in the kitchen.

Tea is not part of God's original diet, however, the consumption of non-caffeine green teas and herbal teas can be excellent sources of antioxidants.

White Flour

Bread has been a staple food from earliest times. Evidence of the use of bread has been found in ancient Egyptian tombs and other human settlements. Both leavened and unleavened bread is mentioned in the Old Testament, and even today, Jews commemorate the Exodus from Egypt by eating unleavened bread.

Ancient ruins of Pompeii and other ruined cities reveal that bakeries existed in historic times. In Rome, around 168BC, a baker's guild was formed with the bakers themselves enjoying special societal privileges open only to freemen of the city.

In early English times, the ruling classes kept the price of bread down for fear of rebellion that often followed famine. King James passed laws in 1202 regulating the price of bread.

The invention of the steam engine and the industrial revolution changed the lives of people in many ways. A Swiss engineer invented a new type of mill using rollers made of steel that operated one on top of the other. The rollers were powered by steam engines and the new method proved so successful that within 30 years, almost all the windmill and watermill driven mills were demolished or abandoned.

Roller milling and sifting technology allowed for the floury portion of the grain to be separated from the outer bran and inner germ. This makes the flour not only whiter, but also able to be stored for longer periods of time. Unfortunately, much of the nutrition comes from the germ and bran. White bread, much beloved by the rich, could now be produced at a much lower price thereby becoming available to everyone.

Today, there are many types of flours, but they can be broadly categorized by their rate of extraction, referring to the percentage of grain that is present in the flour. Three basic categories are (1) wholemeal with 100% retention of the grain which is by far the healthiest and most natural choice, (2) brown with 75 to 80% of the original grain containing some bran and germ, and (3) white with 75% of the wheat grain used containing no bran or germ.

While bread is regarded as the staff of life, modern

white breads, and other products made from white flour, are denuded of much of the benefits of the bran and germ.

Fast Food

Technology has benefited society in many ways and has made our lives easier. Indeed, this book was originally written using a word-processor on a computer, and the Internet was used to assist in research. Unfortunately, in all this convenience of a technologically driven world, it seems that the simple art of making healthy nutritious meals has been abandoned to multi-national food companies and fast food chains primarily driven by the need to make profits and returns to shareholders.

With warm climate and cheap land, the population of Southern California tripled in only a short time, sprawling in all directions. After World War II, Southern California became a rich and prosperous area, with all life revolving around the automobile, all but wiping out tram and train networks. This inspired such innovations as the first motel, the first drive-in bank, the first drive-in movies, even the first drive-in church opened by Robert Schuller preaching on Sunday mornings in a drive-in theatre! Of course, there were also the first drive-in restaurants. These restaurants were often well lit with multi-colored neon signs designed to be easily seen from the road, and hired young girls as waitresses known as carhops. A new culture was born.[20]

In 1937, Richard and Mac McDonald opened a drive-in restaurant. But in 1948, they fired all their carhops and refurbished their restaurant to increase the speed in which food was served. Most foods were eliminated from the menu, and everything that required a knife or fork to eat were removed. They replaced cutlery with paper cups, plates and bags. They were truly the pioneers of today's fast food restaurant concept. They revolutionized the restaurant business forever. The McDonald brother's food was very affordable, and soon families queued up to treat themselves and their children to a restaurant eating experience.

Ray Croc, a traveling salesman, recognized the huge potential of the McDonald bothers "speedee" food concept. In 1954, a deal was struck, and Ray Croc himself opened up a new McDonalds restaurant in Des Plaines in 1955. The McDonalds Corporation was born, and by 1958, 100 million hamburgers were sold. Today McDonalds has over 30,000 restaurants worldwide.[21]

At the age of 65, Harland Sanders used his $105 social security check to start a new business. In 1952, Sanders himself opened the first Kentucky Fried Chicken restaurant, and KFC became one of the largest restaurant chains in the US.[22] The greatest marketing ploy used by KFC is the aura of intrigue surrounding the so-called secret recipe of 11 different herbs and spices.[23]

Fast food restaurant chains promote their food as healthy, but in fact, they often serve food high in fat, sugar and salt, and contain many food additives and artificial flavorings. A popular fast food hamburger contains 560 calories, 16% calories from fat and a whopping 1,070mg of sodium, primarily from salts added to the ingredients.[24]

Consider a typical sample lunch at a fast food restaurant....

Hamburger	560 calories
Large French fries	550 calories
Medium milk shake	720 calories
Total	*1,830 calories*

And that's only one meal! This number of calories is nearly enough for an entire day, so imagine what the total number of calories people are typically eating each day. This number could easily be 3,000 to 4,000 per day, which would require about 3 to 4 hours continuous jogging to burn off, just in order to stop getting fatter. There is absolutely no hope of losing weight under these circumstances.

Scientists have known for a long time that eating less (therefore, lowering calories) results in longer-living animals, sometimes up to 40% longer.[25] Although it remains to be proven that this also applies to humans, it is commonly believed that lowering calories to a sustainable minimum level will assist in slowing down the ageing process. Remember the Hunzakuts introduced in Chapter 1, the group of people who live to over 100 years old without any of today's lifestyle diseases? They eat only about 1,900 calories per day.

The fast food industry has also been disastrous for the environment. Vast amounts of packaging, most of which ends up littering streets and finding its way into waterways. Local councils list fast food packaging as one of the most numerous litter items.[26, 27]

Billions of dollars every year are spent by the fast food industry to advertise directly to children, and this marketing is as strong as ever. The number of television advertisements for fast food a child is likely to see during school holidays...[28]

We have a very unfortunate symbiosis, given that increased watching on TV means increasing exposure to junk-food advertising, thus reinforcing the likelihood of child and adult excessive weight and obesity. The Australian Division of General Practice 2003 study showed that a child watching four hours of TV a day during six weeks of holidays would view 649 junk-food ads, 404 for fast food, 135 for drinks and 44 for ice-cream products. Advertising is an intrinsic and important facet of the market, and it has increased remarkably in its ubiquity and ingenuity to encourage us to consume the new products. [The Age, March 28, 2005]

Fast food companies are notoriously litigious, stopping at nothing to ensure that they and their products are not criticized. The McSpotlight anti-Macdonald's website lists the censorship strategy of the McDonald's corporation against individuals and groups who dare to question the quality of their food.[29]

Food Additives

Scientists have discovered that out of the thousands of chemicals in living cells, some have very specific functions. These active chemicals are now mostly synthesized and used instead of or alongside natural components. Citric acid, for example, used to be extracted from lemons, but is now synthesized in laboratories.

Food additives have been used for centuries, but were primarily restricted to salt, sugar, spices and vinegars. However, a whole new food additive industry has arisen complementing the Golden Age of Food Processing of the 1950's. As a result, there has been a massive increase in the chemical adulteration of food.

Food additive companies continually create new chemicals to manipulate, preserve, and transform our food. These chemicals mimic natural flavors, and color foods to make them look more natural or fresh. They may also preserve foods for longer and longer periods of time. Today, some foods are even made entirely from chemicals such as coffee creamers, sugar substitutes, and candies comprised entirely of artificial ingredients.[30]

Food additives are used for many different purposes, and it is surprising the array of different applications. These include acidity/alkalinity regulators, anti-caking agents, antioxidants, bulking agents, colorings, emulsifiers, firming agents, stabilizers, flavor enhancers, foaming agents, gelling agents, glazing agents, humectants (reduce moisture loss), preservatives, raising agents, sweeteners and thickeners.[31]

However, food additives pose a risk, as explained by the World Health Organization...[32]

Food additives and contaminants resulting from food manufacturing and processing can also adversely affect health. Chemicals are the building blocks of life and affect many, if not all, aspect of human metabolism. However, human exposure to toxic chemicals and nutritional imbalances are currently known or suspected to be responsible for promoting or causing cancer, kidney and liver dysfunction, hormonal imbalance, immune system suppression, musculoskeletal disease, birth defects, premature births, impeded nervous and sensory system development, reproductive disorders, mental health problems, cardiovascular diseases, genitor-urinary disease, old-age dementia, and learning disabilities. [World Health Organization]

The BBC news in the UK reported the effects of food additives on children...[33]

Additives in popular snacks can cause hyper-activity and tantrums in young children, a study suggests. Research carried out by the independent watchdog the Food Commission found that so-called 'E-numbers' may adversely affect one in four toddlers. [BBC

News, 25th October, 2002]

Artificially manufactured chemical food additives are not part of God's original diet, and should be avoided as much as possible. Take for example, a popular cola drink. It contains the following cocktail of chemical additives...

Preservative 211: Sodium Benzoate. Used as a preservative but only effective in acidic environments such as soft drinks. May cause allergic reactions and is not recommended for consumption by children.

Color E150d: Caramel. This food coloring ranges from dark brown to black and is manufactured by heating sugar with ammonia and sulphites.

Food Acid E330: Citric Acid. The most widely used organic food acid. Occurs naturally in citrus fruits but may also be prepared from the fermentation of molasses. It is a colorless, crystalline compound belonging to the family of carboxylic acids, and is used as an antioxidant, preservative and acid regulator.

Food Acid E338: Phosphoric Acid: Used as a rust remover, in detergents and a metal treatment. Impure phosphoric acid is used as a fertilizer. Gives soft drinks their sharp taste.

Sweetener E950: Acesulphane Potassium. 200 times sweeter than sugar, and has a bitter after taste. Used widely as artificial sweetener in low joule gums, drinks, diet foods, etc. It is a possible carcinogen in humans.

Sweetener E951: Aspartame. An intense sweetener synthesized from aspartic acid and phenylalanine. It is about 200 times sweeter than sugar by weight. Aspartame was originally banned as a carcinogenic but is now allowed. It is possibly one of the most controversial food additives on the market due to so much conflicting research.

Phenylalanine: An essential amino acid found in proteins, but when isolated and added as a food additive, can act as a neurotoxin and may damage neurons in the brain.[34]

Caffeine: One of the world's most popular drugs alongside nicotine and alcohol. When isolated, caffeine is a white crystalline powder and tastes very bitter. It is used as a cardiac stimulant and as a mild diuretic, but mostly, it is used to provide a boost of energy or a sense of heightened awareness. Caffeine is a very addictive drug, and operates in the same manner as amphetamines, cocaine, and heroine used to stimulate the brain.

Is this what God intended us to eat when He planted the garden in Eden?

Chapter 4
OTHER IMPORTANT FACTORS

As we have seen, the food we eat has a very significant impact on our health and general well-being. However, there are a number of other significant and important factors that contribute to our health, as well. All these, as a complete package, provide us with optimal conditions for maintaining excellent health throughout our entire lives.

Water, Humble H_2O

Water is a chemical compound comprised of atoms from two very explosive gasses: oxygen and hydrogen. Two very light hydrogen atoms are attached to each heavier oxygen atom, giving water the familiar chemical formula H_2O.

Water, comprising some 75% of the earth's surface, is a very stable, virtually indestructible and unique substance. It can exist in solid, liquid and gaseous states. Humans cannot survive for more than a few days without it.

Of all the water contained in the earth, 97.5% is salty and therefore cannot be readily used. Of the remaining 2.5%, approximately three quarters is locked up in polar ice caps, soil moisture, aquifers and ground water. Only about 0.01% of the earth's water is available from lakes, rivers, reservoirs and underground sources that can be tapped.[1] Even so, much of this water is not utilized due to inaccessibility, transportation difficulties, climatic conditions, political tensions or lack of money for development. The net result is that the actual percentage of water directly available for human use is very small indeed.

Since ancient days, the control of water for crops and human consumption has been of vital concern. With some 70 to 75% of human water usage required for irrigation and agriculture, and 20% for industrial and urban purposes,[2] it is no surprise that drought has been the causes of whole civilizations collapsing. Even today, drought seriously affects a nation's GDP and threatens economic prosperity. Almost all the world's nations are considered vulnerable to water scarcity.

Water has been used in judgment, danger and death, such as the Great Flood of Noah and the drowning of Egyptians in the Red Sea. Good rainfall is a sign of God's favor, and God even describes himself as living water…

> **Those who depart from Me shall be written in the earth, because they have forsaken the Lord, the fountain of living waters. Jeremiah 17:13**

And of course, the water that Jesus gives will ensure that nobody thirsts…

> **Whoever drinks of the water that I shall give him will never thirst. But the water that I shall give him will become in him a fountain of water springing up into everlasting life. John 4:14**

Jesus himself was baptized in water, exemplifying the important connection between water and human existence, judgment and repentance.

Water Pollution

While water itself is a very stable chemical compound, it is very easily polluted. It is estimated that 80% of infectious diseases today are caused by waterborne infections or by diseases where water plays a significant role. Third-world countries are particularly vulnerable.[3]

According to the World Health Organization, waterborne diseases are the leading cause of disease and death in the world with 3.4 million people dying per annum, including 4,000 children per day. These diseases include diarrhea, ascariasis (intestinal worm infection), filariasis (round worm infection), schistosomiasis (schistosoma parasite), malaria (plasmodium parasite), dengue fever (infection from mosquito bites), cholera (small intestine infection from cholorea bacteria), amongst many others.[4]

One of the plagues of Egypt was the pollution of water...

> **So he lifted up the rod and struck the waters that were in the river, in the sight of Pharoah and the sight of his servants. And all the waters that were in the river were turned to blood. The fish that were in the river died, the river stank, and the Egyptians could not drink the water of the river. Exodus 7:20-21**

And when the Isrealites were finally free from their Egyptian oppressors, they wandered through the Wilderness of Shur, finding no water. After three days, they came to Marah, only to find that the water there was polluted...

> **Now when they came to Marah, they could not drink the waters of Marah, for they were bitter. Therefore, the name of it was called Marah. Exodus 15:23**

At least a third of the world's population lacks safe,

clean water due to pollution caused by industrial and domestic dumping directly into rivers and lakes. Even today, industries in Western societies still continue to dump toxic wastes into waterways and oceans.

Agricultural runoff also threatens the world's drinking supply. Urine, fecal material, toxic herbicides, pesticides and a myriad of other chemicals enter waterways by surface runoff or direct discharge.

Poisons Added to Water

While water is very vulnerable to all sorts of pollution, further assault is made to public water supplies through fluoridation, chlorination and other chemical processes.

The story of fluoridation goes back to 1850, when it was discovered that fluoride emissions from iron, copper and aluminum foundries were poisoning livestock and crops.[5] By the turn of the century, lawsuits threatened the smelting industry, and in the 1920's, fluoride emissions were out of control. In 1930 a major air pollution disaster occurred in Belgium, where fluoride poisoning caused the death of 60 people.[6]

By the late 1930's, when gearing up for war, the aluminum industry was producing unprecedented volumes of sodium fluoride waste. In 1939, the first proposal to fluoridate water was made in the US. This proposal came not from doctors, dentists or other health professionals, but by aluminum companies threatened by fluoride damage claims.[7] By the 1950's, fluoridation of drinking water was widespread practice in many countries. However, fluoride is a serious poison, and so fluoridated water should never be consumed.

And it seems that incidence of tooth cavities in fluoridated communities is not different to non-fluoridated communities. The good news is that, despite pressure from dental organizations, many countries have now banned fluoridation for environmental, health, legal or ethical reasons. These countries include China, Austria, Belgium, Finland, Germany, Denmark, Norway, Sweden, Holland, Hungary and Japan.[8]

Chlorine's disinfectant properties were known as early as the 1840's, where it was used in Austrian maternity wards to prevent infection following the birth of babies. In 1905, chlorine was added to London's water supply which did result in a significant diminishing of a typhoid epidemic. By World War I, chlorine's use as a drinking water disinfectant was widespread.

Unfortunately, although it helps to reduce water borne bacteria that causes disease, water chlorination suffers from a number of drawbacks. Chlorine destroys much of the friendly intestinal bacteria that are responsible for digestion of food and absorption of important vitamins such as vitamin B_{12}.

Chlorine itself can combine with organic matter in water to form organochlorides. These organochlorides do not degrade very well and are stored in the body's fatty tissue. Chlorine also aggravates asthma and increases the risk of cancer, amongst many other risks. To make matters worse, inhaling chlorine released during hot showers can be many times greater than actually drinking chlorinated water.[9]

But fluorine and chlorine are not the only chemicals added to water...[10]

> *In the USA, Ralph Nader's Center for Responsive Law found more that 2000 toxic chemicals in drinking water, of which less than 30 are tested for or monitored. So there are limits to the quality of water we can expect to receive from municipal authorities. [John Archer]*

These chemicals include sodium silicofluoride, fluo-rosilicic acid, sodium hypochlorite, lime (calcium oxide and calcium hydroxide) and alum (potassium aluminum sulphate). Also added to water are pH adjusters, dispersants to prevent crystal precipitation, sequestering agents to prevent absorption of minerals, oxidizing agents such as potassium permanganate to neutralize reducing agents, and reducing agents such as sodium metabisulfite to neutralize oxidizing agents.[11]

Indeed, the number of chemicals that can be legally added to drinking water is astonishingly high...[12]

> *Up to fifty different chemicals can be legally added to our water in order to 'purify' it. [John Archer]*

So, is tap water good water? Emphatically, the answer is No! Apart from the chemical onslaught described above, water also passes through various filtering and chemical processes. These processes can be categorized as follows...

Screen Purification: Coarse screening removes large particulate matter at the source of intake to prevent damage and clogging of equipment downstream.

Clarification: Includes the addition of chemical coagulants and pH adjustment chemicals that react to form floc, which settles in settling tanks or is removed through gravity filters.

Lime Treatment: Lime and soda ash is added to reduce the level of calcium and magnesium, and is referred to as lime softening.

Disinfection: After water has been clarified and softened, chlorine gas is fed into the water to kill bacteria. Chlorine levels must be constantly monitored to ensure so-called safe levels.

pH Adjustment: The pH of the water is adjusted so that it falls within a range of 7.5 to 8.0 in order to prevent erosion of pipes, and in particular, to stop lead entering the water supply.

This chemically laden and ultra treated water is then pumped through municipal pipe systems that can sometimes be over 100 years old. These pipes contain iron, lead, copper, brass and other metallic elements that water inevitably absorbs in its long journey to our homes. Once the water reaches our homes, it is at the mercy of the quality of the pipes, taps and plumbing within the home. It may look clean, but it is a veritable cocktail of dangerous chemical elements and compounds.

Water in the Body

The human body is comprised of 70% water. In fact, water is an essential fluid involved in the mechanics and chemistry of every function of the body. Water lost through perspiration, exhalation and urination must be continuously replaced. Fortunately, the body has a wonderful mechanism called thirst to make us want to drink water, when even just a 2% drop in water levels can trigger signs of dehydration.

As the body has no use for inorganic elements and compounds such as calcium carbonate (the active ingredient in cement that makes it harden), it must attempt to get rid of these inorganic compounds in any way possible. Calcium deposits form in various places, causing the formation of stones in organs such as the gall bladder and kidneys, gout in the feet, arthritis and rheumatism in the joints, and hardening of the arteries.

It should be noted that it is not water's role to furnish our bodies with minerals it uses for regeneration and replenishment. This comes from the food we eat. Water's role is to aid digestion and elimination, regulate body temperature, provide lubrication for joint surfaces, form the base for saliva, provide a detoxifying agent, and regulate metabolism.[13]

When we drink, water is absorbed through the large intestines and is distributed for use within the cells (intracellular) and between the cells and bloodstream (extracellular). Intracellular and extracellular water passes freely between each other via cell membranes, but substances dissolved in water cannot easily pass through. If we consume very salty food, the blood will contain excessive concentrations of salt, causing water to be drawn out of the cells, whereby the cells actually shrink in size, a process known as cellular dehydration, a stimulus for thirst.[14]

So important is the role of water in the economy of the body that a consistent lack of it can be a cause of many illnesses. Dr F. Batmanghelidj, MD, describes how symptoms of sickness are actually due to the body signaling for more water...[15]

With the appearance of these signals, the body should be provided with water for the rationing systems to distribute. However, medical practitioners have been taught to silence these signals with chemical products. Of course, they have zero understanding of the significance of this most gross error. The various signals produced by these water distributors are indicators of regional thirst and drought in the body. At the onset, they can be relieved by an increased intake of water itself, yet they are improperly dealt with by the use of commercial chemical products until pathology is established and diseases are born. It is unfortunate that this mistake is continued until the use of more and more chemicals to treat the developing symptoms and complications of dehydration becomes unavoidable, and then the patient dies. [Dr F. Batmanghelidj]

Water is therefore the cheapest and most readily available medicine for a dehydrated body. I remember when I presented to hospital with diabetes, I was so dehydrated that I took in nearly two bags of saline intravenous drip!

Our bodies require between 1 and 2 liters of water per day, depending on activity levels. But poor sources of water include sodas, manufactured beverages, and caffeine drinks such as coffee and tea. While these drinks contain water, they do not adequately serve the body's need for water.

These beverages contain caffeine and sugar, with all the addictive properties of a drug. Indeed, many people who give up drinking colas, coffee or tea report withdrawal symptoms such as headaches, dizziness, nervousness and the like. It is unfortunate that most people require caffeine pick-me-up's in the morning in an effort to wake them up. But this boost is borrowed energy that must be later replenished, or until the next cup of coffee, in which case more energy is borrowed again. Many people continue this vicious up-and-down cycle of caffeine stimulant input and depressive lack of energy day-by-day, year-by-year.

Distilled Water

Ideally, water should be odorless, colorless and tasteless, and (by definition) have a pH level of 7, neither acidic nor alkaline.

Not all water is the same, as all water suffers from various concentrations of impurities and chemicals. The exception, however, is STEAM DISTILLED water. This is water that has been boiled to produce steam, and the steam condensed into the purest water possible. Distillation, together with a final carbon filter, totally removes all bacteria and viruses, infused gasses such as chlorine, fluorine and radon, and compounds such as detergents, phosphates, pesticides, herbicides, sulfates and chlorides. Metals such as cadmium, calcium, lead, magnesium, iron, copper, aluminum, mercury, zinc (in fact, almost every metal in the periodic table can be found in water, even uranium), are also removed.

When distilled water is used for drinking and cooking, it reaches the liver already in the purest state possible, giving the liver a much-reduced workload. Once water is purified by the liver, it is passed into the bloodstream, lymph system, intestines and other areas for use. Purified water, a natural and powerful solvent, is used to collect and remove debris and minerals rejected or spent by the cells of the body.

Steam distilled water is by far the best option. A household distiller can be purchased for around $400 to $1,000 providing cheap on-going quality water for both drinking and cooking. Filtered water, water purified by reverse osmosis, or bottled water, should only be consumed in emergencies when distilled water is not available.

Dr Allen Banik, MD, an expert in the application of water in medicine, says that about distilled water...[16]

As distilled water enters the body, it again picks up mineral deposits accumulated in the joints, and begins to carry them out. Gall stones and kidney stones get smaller and smaller until they can safely pass out through their ducts. Little by little, arthritic pains become less as joints become more elastic as blood pressures tend to become more normal. Gradually the outlook on life becomes a little more youthful...while the squeaking rocking chair will give way to the web covered golf clubs. [Dr Allen Banik]

Bottled spring water is expensive and the cost of buying it can easily be recouped by purchasing a distiller, where the purest water can be made for only a few cents per liter. The source, quality and processing of bottled water can be questionable as more and more companies clamor for the lucrative bottled water market.

A diet high in fresh plant foods is naturally also high in water purified by the plants themselves. This makes dehydration most unlikely on the Genesis diet, particularly if one or two liters of pure distilled water daily are also consumed.

Fruit & Vegetable Juicing

Aircraft run most efficiently on fuels they have been designed to use. If automobile fuel is used in a light aircraft designed to run on avgas, the aircraft's engine may turn over, but it will splutter, knock and misfire. It will certainly not provide enough thrust to fly the aircraft, and no pilot in their right mind would try. Eventually, the engine will be ruined, and will need to be replaced at huge expense.

Our bodies function at maximum efficiency when fueled properly. This fuel is predominately complex carbohydrates, but also includes proteins, amino acids, fats and enzymes supplied by fruits, vegetables, legumes and whole grains obtained in the Genesis Diet. Even so, today's nutrient depleted soils and modern sowing, harvesting and processing methods mean that different fruits and vegetables from different geographical locations will have varying degrees of nutrient content. One way of ensuring a plentiful supply of highly absorbable nutrients is to drink fresh fruit and vegetable juices.

By separating the minerals and distilled water from the plant pulp, nutrients are assimilated into the body very quickly. Another major benefit of drinking fresh vegetable juices is the presence of nutritional enzymes, the life-force found in raw, uncooked food. Enzymes act as catalysts in chemical reactions but do not in themselves alter chemically. Fresh, raw vegetable juicing is like taking a natural multi-vitamin and mineral tonic. Drinking juices daily will greatly improve general health and the ability to fight off diseases.

Dr Norman Walker, DSc, who introduced the world to vegetable juicing in the early 1900's, has this to say about the benefits of fresh juices...[17]

> *The juices extracted from fresh-raw vegetables and fruits are the means by which we can furnish all the cells and tissues of the body with the elements and the nutritional enzymes they need in the manner they can be most readily digested and assimilated. [Dr Norman Walker]*

The juice of carrots can be consumed on its own or as a base for mixing with other vegetable juices. These juices contain beta-carotenes, B-complex vitamins, vitamins C, D, E, G and K, as well as minerals such as sodium, potassium, calcium, magnesium and iron. Juices also contain all eight essential amino acids.

Fresh juice is far superior to the commercial bottled or canned varieties. These go through a number of processes including pasteurization (heating the juice to very high temperatures), which destroys the enzymes and minerals contained in the juice. To add insult, these juices may then be artificially colored, flavored, reconstituted and chemically treated.

Juices are not a concentrated food. Indeed, juices contain mostly purified water of the highest quality with nutrients in comparatively small volume. But it is this small volume of nutrients that are very beneficial to the cells of the body.

Fasting

No doubt, eating is a pleasure and enjoyment given to us from God, who gave us a wide variety of edible plants and great tasting fruits for us to enjoy.

> **Here is what I have seen: It is good and fitting that for one to eat and drink, and to enjoy the good of all his labor in which he toils under the sun all the days of his life which God gives him; for it is his heritage. Ecclesiastes 5:18**

Food brings Christians together, as part of fellowship and worship, with thanksgiving for being blessed by Him.

> **When you have eaten and are full, then you shall bless the Lord your God for the good land which He has given you. Deuteronomy 8:10**

And there will come a time when we will be invited to a banquet at the marriage supper of the Lamb...

> **Then he said to me, Write: Blessed are those who are called to the marriage supper of the Lamb! Revelation 19:9**

Yet God has a place for fasting in our lives, too. The word "fasting" comes from the Hebrew nesteia, a concatenation of ne (negative) and esthio (to eat). Thus fasting simply means "not to eat." Unfortunately, fasting is not practiced extensively in modern western Christianity, and indeed, the concept seems almost foreign to us.

There are many examples of fasting in the Old and New Testaments. Moses performed the first recorded fast in the Bible...

> **When I went up into the mountain to receive the tablets of stone, the tablets of the covenant which the Lord made with you, then I stayed on the mountain forty days and forty nights. I neither ate bread nor drank water. Deuteronomy 9:9**

The household of Esther fasted for three days in order to help the Jews...

> **Go, gather all the Jews who are present in Shushan, and fast for me; neither eat nor drink for three days, night or day. My maids and I will fast likewise. And so I will go to the king, which is against the law; and if I perish, I perish! Esther 4:16**

Jesus himself fasted often, once for a total of 40 days. No wonder that "afterward He was hungry"! (Matthew 4:1). Fasting is a powerful weapon in the Christian's armor, and an expression of spiritual warfare, wholeheartedness, repentance and obedience...

> **Now therefore, says the Lord, turn to Me with all your heart, with fasting, with weeping, and with mourning. Joel 2:12**

The Bible has many more examples of fasting for reasons of victory in war (Judges 20:26), repentance (1 Samuel 7:6), mourning (1 Kings 21:27), overcoming demonic strongholds (Mark 9:29) and an attribute of ministry (2 Corinthians 6:5). Whatever the reason for fasting, it will be rewarded...

But you, when you fast, anoint your head and wash your face, so that you do not appear to men to be fasting, but to your Father who is in the secret place, and your Father who sees in secret will reward you openly. Matthew 6:17-18

God would not require us to fast if fasting was dangerous or injurious to our health. Indeed, fasting is literally a doctor waiting to help us. It gives our bodies a rest from the enormous task of digesting food, and allows it to begin the process of cleansing out toxins and other debris. It is the great cleanser and purifier.

Those who practice fasting on a regular basis say that it keeps them sharp and alert, and contrary to what many may think, actually helps to increase athletic performance. Sporting performance can be enhanced as the body does not need to direct energy into digesting food, although very strenuous exercise during a fast is not recommended.

Why do we shun food when we are sick? This is a natural response of the body, saying to itself: "I am sick. I need to cleanse myself of toxins that are causing sickness. I do not wish to eat now, because I need the energy to deal with it." Also, notice when we go through emotional trauma or time of mourning, we often do not feel like eating.

Like prayer, fasting is personal. However, fasting at least once a week for 24 or 36 hours is most beneficial. During a fast, be certain to drink enough pure, distilled water and/or vegetable juices to avoid dehydration and facilitate the cleansing process. Longer fasts of 2 or 3 days can be attempted every 3 months or so, while even longer fasts may need proper supervision.

Fasting, however, is not always pleasant, and is a discipline that must be practiced. First of all, of course, we get hungry. Then the tongue will develop an unpleasant coating. Other maladies that may arise include bad breath, body odor, skin eruptions, nausea, darkened urine, headaches and accelerated mucous drainage. All these symptoms, however, are due to the body eliminating toxins.

As the body becomes more and more chemically balanced after a period of eating a plant-based Genesis diet, fasting becomes easier and the symptoms less severe. The results, however, are worth it as our bodies become better cleansed internally.

Exercise Turn Fat to Fit

Proper diet and regular exercise is the best combination for maximum weight loss and health maintenance. The importance of exercise cannot be over-emphasized — it is an extremely important part of our daily health program. Exercise helps to lower blood pressure, regulate blood sugar levels and tone the body's muscles. It increases the body's rate of metabolism even higher, burning calories faster.

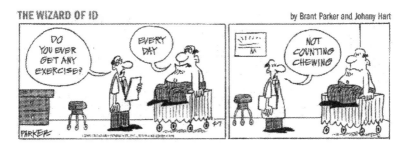

© Creators Syndicate, Inc. Reprinted by permission of John L. Hart FLP and Creators Syndicate, Inc

Walking is the best exercise, does not cost any money, can be performed anywhere and at anytime, and is very low impact and safe to do. It is the most natural exercise.

It is more likely that walking will be maintained over a longer period of time than other exercises. Brisk walking burns about 420 calories per hour, so a good 1 hour walk will burn about 1/5 or 1/6 of our daily calorie intake. Unless you are a serious athlete or extremely fit, it is unlikely that you would jog for an hour. Briskly walking uphill burns nearly as many calories as jogging, anyway, so try to plan walks to include inclines and hills.

But walking has many more benefits than just burning calories. For a start, walking tones most muscles in the body such as calf's, tibias anteriors (shin), hamstrings, quadriceps, hip flexors, buttocks, abdominals, arms and shoulders. This muscle tone gives the body shape making you look good.

Walking also builds aerobic capacity. The sustained, repeated, rhythmic working out of the large muscle groups also strengthens the heart and lungs. Long term aerobic conditioning has many benefits including protection against heart disease and stroke. Walking combats high blood pressure, diabetes, and also wards off osteoporosis due to the strengthening of bones and increasing bone mass. Regular walking helps keep the bowels regular and prevents constipation.

Walking generates an overall feeling of well-being, and can relieve depression, anxiety, and stress by producing endorphins, the body's natural tranquilizer. A brisk walk will relax you and stimulate your thinking.

In addition to a healthy regime of walking, taking up a sport such as golf, cycling, swimming or some other aerobic sport will add the fun factor to your exercise regime. Playing competitive sport ensures that you exercise regularly and vigorously, raising a good sweat while enjoying yourself. Joining a sporting club can also be a great social outlet, too.

Occasional weight and resistance training is also beneficial. A set of barbell weights is not expensive and can easily be used indoors or outdoors. Weight and other resistance training such as push-ups and chin-ups build up muscle and body tone while helping to get rid of that unwanted flab.

If you are overweight, have medical problems, or have

not exercised for a long time, it is far better to initially concentrate on diet and safely perform a moderate amount of exercise. As the weeks and months go by, you will begin to lose weight and feel lighter, healthier and more energetic. At this point, you can increase your exercise regime gradually until you are comfortable with a daily routine.

The secret is to not become overly obsessive with exercise, where too much can be just as harmful as too little. For example, jogging multiplies the body's weight on the ankles, knees and lower back, causing a detrimental effect on the skeleton and joints.

> **For bodily exercise profits a little, but godliness is profitable for all things, having promise of the life that now is and of that which is to come. 1 Timothy 4:8**

Timothy wrote this at a time when there were no cars, buses, trains and airplanes. It was a time when people did mainly manual work and walked everywhere they wanted to go. They were already getting sufficient exercise in their daily routine, and so additional exercise was not warranted, and such time was better spent concentrating on godliness and serving the Lord.

Indeed, it is only in the last one hundred years or so that widespread surface, sea and air transportation has made it possible to travel both short and long distances without any major effort. Even as little as sixty years ago, few would have thought that we would one day be able to cross the Atlantic Ocean in only just eight hours sitting in relative comfort, or travel from one side of the continent to the other in just five. We even have moving walkways in airports to make it easier for us!

Oxygen, Sunshine and Rest

Fill your lungs with life-sustaining oxygen by practicing deep breathing. If necessary, make frequent trips to the country just to breathe in the crisp air. Combined with vigorous walking, you have achieved the best of both worlds!

The sun is your friend, not your enemy. The sun's solar energy is a primary source of vitamin D and its soothing rays brings relaxation and peacefulness. Gentle sunbaths in the early morning and late afternoon (thereby avoiding the harsh midday sun), bring immense health benefits.

In our modern world, we seem to be trying to do more and more, constantly pushing our bodies to the limit. Proper rest and sleep is vitally important — they revitalize the body.

Chapter 5
LIVESTOCK REVOLUTION

The Livestock Revolution is a term applied to the recent explosion in the population of livestock on the earth, particularly in developing countries.[1] This explosion is growing faster than the human population.[2]

The estimated global livestock and avian population today is 20 billion head of livestock and 15.7 billion fowl, representing a 60% and 400% increase respectively since 1961.[3] This represents populations thousands of times greater than what would occur if these animals were left to live and breed in their natural environments. For example, in the United States, there is an estimated 6.4 million wild turkeys,[4] while 400 million farmed turkeys are eaten annually.[5]

Over 10 billion animals were slaughtered for food in the United States in 2001, excluding fish and other aquatic life. Of these 10 billion, 8.9 billion were chickens, with the largest chicken processor, Tyson Foods, slaughtering 2.2 billion.[6] When these animals are slaughtered, they do not just queue up meekly to die.

Even the lovable and gentle guinea pig is farmed for food, animal experiments and testing of cosmetics, toiletries and cleaning products. In Peru, 65 million guinea pigs are slaughtered every year for food.[7]

As Christians, we believe in Jesus and confess that He is Lord in order to be spared from an eternity in the lake of fire, forever separated from God. We are created in the image of God, and Jesus died to save our sins. In this sense, God considers man to be of more value than animals...

Do not fear, therefore; you are of more value than many sparrows. Luke 12:7

While all animals have their own instincts and intelligences, they do not have souls that require redemption, and so they do not go to hell. Even so, God does not allow animals to die apart from His will...

Your righteousness is like the great mountains; Your judgments are a great deep; O Lord, You preserve man and beast. Psalm 36:6

And not one of them falls to the ground apart from your Father's will. Matthew 10:29

Thus, animals should only die in the will of God, and not at the behest of man for the purpose of profit or even in the name of advancement of science. This is why God originally gave man benevolent stewardship (dominion) over all the animals of the land, in the air, and in the sea. We therefore should value the beauty and interdependence of flora and fauna in the natural world that God created.

Indeed, animals are capable of praising God...

Praise the Lord from the earth, you great sea creatures and all the depths. Psalm 148:7

Let everything that has breath praise the Lord. Psalm 150:6

This is not to say that animals should be totally left

alone. Remember that God brought every animal to Adam to see what he would name them (Genesis 2:19), thus establishing a loving relationship with them. The entire works of God, including animals, were created for us...

> **You made him to have dominion over the works of Your hands; You have put all things under his feet, all sheep and oxen, even beasts of the fields, the birds of the air, and the fish of the sea that pass through the paths of the seas. Psalm 8:6-8**

Cruelty to animals for cruelty's sake, the hunting of animals for pleasure and sport, the exploitation of animals in high-density factory farms and testing of cosmetics and other products on animals should therefore be abhorred by Christians.

> **A righteous man regards the life of his animal. Proverbs 12:10**

So what right do we have to treat animals with such cruelty and indifference when...

> **The Lord is good to all, and His tender mercies are over all His works. Psalm 145:9**

The prophet Isaiah describes a new creation where man and animals will live together in harmony, and there will be no eating of animal flesh...

> **The wolf also shall dwell with the lamb, the leopard shall lie down with the young goat, the calf and the young lion and the fatling together, and a little child shall lead them. The cow and the bear shall graze, their young ones shall lie down together, and the lion shall eat straw like an ox. Isaiah 11:6-7**

> **The wolf and the lamb shall feed together, the lion shall eat straw like the ox, and dust shall be the serpent's food. They shall not hurt nor destroy in all My holy mountain, says the Lord. Isaiah 65:25**

This new heaven, new earth and New Jerusalem will come after the tribulation period described in the book of Revelation, when perfection will be re-established.

In the parable of the lost sheep in Matthew chapter 18, Jesus tells the story of a man with 100 sheep, but one of them goes astray. The shepherd leaves the 99 and searches for the single lost sheep. In John chapter 10, Jesus describes Himself as the Good Shepherd, because He knows His sheep, and His sheep know Him. These metaphors were used by Jesus because the people would understand and relate the love of God to His people in terms of the love a shepherd has for his sheep, as was the custom at the time.

But the current cruel methods of factory farming animals are so far removed from Biblical principles that it could not be called husbandry at all, as we shall see.

Kentucky Fried Misery

Chickens are intelligent birds that have a complex social structure. God created them to nest, roost, and root in the ground for their food. A mother hen takes care of her chicks with the love and attention God programmed in her genetic makeup. Jesus compared His love of Jerusalem to the love of a hen to its chicks…

> **Oh Jerusalem, Jerusalem, the one who kills the prophets and stones those who are sent to her! How often I wanted to gather your children together, as a hen gathers her brood under her wings, but you are not willing! Luke 13:34**

With a growing number of people switching from red meat to poultry in the mistaken belief that chicken is healthier, the chicken industry is booming. These proud birds are crammed by the thousands into battery cages, hardly able to move. For example, poultry get a paltry 600 sq cm per bird (not much larger than the page you are reading now).[8]

Deprived of their natural urges while packed into their cages, chickens begin to peck each other, so much so that the number of deaths caused by this behavior is of concern to the chicken industry. But this concern is not for the welfare of the chickens. Rather, the concern is for the welfare of the bottom line. So, instead of giving the birds more room and providing more humane conditions, the chickens simply have their beaks cut off.[9, 10]

> *It's a damn shame when they kill each other*
> *[referring to chickens pecking each other]. It*
> *means we wasted all the feed that went into*
> *the damn thing. [Herbert Reed]*

Chickens raised for meat (known as broilers), are fed all sorts of growth hormones, antibiotics and other chemicals to make them grow as fast as possible and encourage higher productivity and birth rates through artificial insemination.[11] One study showed that the concentration of arsenic in chickens was up to 9 times the Environment Protection Agency's limit.[12] Often they grow so rapidly that their hearts and lungs are not developed enough, and their legs often cannot support the additional weight. They literally buckle under their own weight.[13]

In the slaughterhouse, chickens suffer immeasurably. Fully conscious birds are hung by their feet in shackles on a moving rail that passes through mechanical blades designed to slit their throats. Unfortunately, many birds are not killed by this method, and once they reach the scalding tank, those that are still alive are boiled live. Chickens normally live up to 10 years, but today they are slaughtered when only about 7 weeks old, essentially when they are still baby birds but double the weight of chicks reared naturally.[14]

Layer hens confined to battery cages supply some 95% of eggs consumed in the western world. The floors of these cages are made of wire and are slanted, causing sever discomfort. Upon hatching, male chickens are of no use, so they are simply put into plastic bags and suffocated or shunted off to become broilers.[15] After a laying cycle, hens are shocked into another laying cycle as quickly as possible. This continuous cycle of laying more and more eggs per bird causes mineral depletion and osteoporosis, with many dying from a condition known as layer fatigue.[16]

A famous libel case is the so-called McLibel trial. This was the British court case between McDonalds and two individuals, Helen Steel and Dave Morris, who distributed a leaflet entitled "What's Wrong With McDonalds? — Everything You Don't Want to Know." The case ran for 2½ years, the longest libel trial in British history, ending in June, 1997. In a two-hour open court reading, Justice Bell said...[17]

> *Nevertheless in my JUDGEMENT the restriction of movement of laying hens throughout their lives in the U.K. and the U.S., and of broiler chickens in their last days in the U.K. and the U.S., and of some sows for virtually the whole of their lives in the U.K. is quite enough to justify the first particular charge of culpable responsibility for cruel practices in the way some of the animals spend their lives. Although not all the particular charges are justified, in my overall JUDGEMENT those that are justified, relating to the restriction of movement*

of battery hens, broiler chickens and chickens who have their throats cut while still fully conscious are sufficient to justify the general charge that the First and Second Plaintiffs are culpably responsible for cruel practices in the rearing and slaughter of some of the animals which are used to produce their food. [Justice Bell]

If all this shocks the reader, then unfortunately it is the sad truth. What a disgrace that modern man pursues profit without even a thought given to the God-given edict of kind stewardship over animals.

So influential are the major fast-food companies, that food processors breed chickens with specific attributes. Eric Schlosser describes one such travesty like this…[18]

The initial test-marketing of McNuggets was so successful that McDonalds enlisted another company, Tyson Foods, to guarantee an adequate supply. Based in Arkansas, Tyson was one of the nation's leading chicken processors, and it soon developed a new breed of chicken to facilitate the production of McNuggets. Dubbed "Mr McDonald," the new breed had unusually large breasts.

There is still a shred of hope, however. One company in Europe is experimenting with more humane free-range environments, and even experimenting with toys hanging from the ceiling, straw bails, wooden perches, and gradual darkness to mimic night and day. All this results in more robust birds, with greater strength and lower mortality rate.[19]

Swine Anguish

Of course, it's not just chickens that are made to suffer. Pigs also suffer horribly. Indeed, pigs are genuinely friendly, affectionate animals and are in every way as intelligent as dogs. Unfortunately, these wonderful creatures are also forced to live their entire lives in cages so narrow that they can't even turn around. Pregnant sows are held in small crates only inches wider than their bodies for weeks at a time. The poor sow cannot sit down and allow the piglets to suckle once they are born.[20]

Apart from living in cramped conditions all their lives, pigs' cages contain wire floors to allow waste to drop through. Unfortunately, this causes the animal extreme discomfort and numerous deformities, but that does not upset the factory pig farmers one bit, it is a matter of business...[21]

> *We don't get paid for producing animals with good posture around here. We get paid by the pound! [J. Messersmith]*

Now, what happens when 80,000 pigs confined to a factory farm urinate and defecate into pits under their cages? The resultant stench is unbearable from the ammonia and methane gases produced. The pigs cannot escape these fumes, and become ill or die due to continuous exposure. Their waste is equivalent to a city of 160,000 people.[22]

Animal industries show appalling disregard for the welfare of their animals by keeping them barely alive until slaughter time. The animals are regarded as mere commodities and hence any cruel practice that improves the bottom line is acceptable...[23]

> *Forget the pig is an animal. Treat him just like a machine in a factory. Schedule treatments*

*like you would lubrication, breeding season
like the first step in an assembly line. And
marketing like the delivery of finished goods.
[J. Byrnes]*

Bovine Agony

Veal calves are a by-product of the dairy industry. Since male calves are of no use to the dairy industry, they are raised for beef or veal. Called early separation, veal cows are taken away almost immediately from their mothers. The baby calves are then fed a diet deficient in iron to keep the flesh white and anemic. This apparently makes veal flesh more appealing to the consumer.[24]

On top of this, veal calves are confined to cramped cages or crates, just like pigs. They are chained so that movement is severely restricted in order to keep the meat tender so muscles are not given a chance to develop. At approximately 16 weeks of age, the weak veal calves are slaughtered.[25]

Dairy cows do not fair much better. Obsessed with increasing milk yield from each cow, the dairy industry simply regards their cows as machines to produce milk, with many being raised in intensive confinement.

To achieve these increased yields, cows are continuously and artificially impregnated. The uterus of the cow is prepared with progesterone, a hormone primarily used for pregnancy maintenance. Pfizer, makers of the EAZI-BREED cattle insert says that with their product "You can start breeding programs at any stage of the estrous cycle. This gives you a new solution for synchronization in heifers."[26]

Dairy cows are milked far more frequently than they ever have been in the past, sometimes up to six times per day (known as 6X). They are fed a concentrated diet of grains rather than natural grasses they were created to eat, selectively bred to increase udder size, and administered with drugs such as Bovine Growth Hormone (BGH) and antibiotics.[27] To the dairy industry, increasing milking frequency is simply an economic measure...[28]

> *Increasing the frequency of milk removal increases milk production in cattle as it does in many species. This is a common management approach to maximize production per cow and to fully optimize capital investment in machinery and facilities. One obvious drawback is the increase in variable costs, mainly labor, required to reap the higher milk yield. [Journal of Dairy Science]*

All this stress on cows significantly affects their health, resulting in painful udder infections and lame and swollen joints. Such cows can no longer support their own weight and simply fall to the ground (known as downed cows). The meat from downed cows was mostly ground into hamburger mince, although after the Mad Cow Disease scare, downed cows are no longer processed for human food.[29]

Mad Cow Disease, properly called Bovine Spongiform Encephalopathy (BSE), is a progressive, degenerative and fatal disease of the central nervous system of cattle. It is believed to be caused by infectious forms of proteins called prions, normally found in animals. It causes the brain to turn into a sponge like consistency. Symptoms of the disease include nervousness, twitching and involuntary muscle movement eventually leading to the inability to stand up. The disease can be transferred to other species, even humans, where it is called Creutzfeldt-Jakob Disease.[30]

The whole debacle of Mad Cow Disease was a disaster waiting to happen. Factory farmed animals reared in restrictive pens are fed hormones, antibiotics and other chemicals to fatten them up quickly. Forever focused on cutting costs, ranchers began to feed their vegetarian animals with ground up diseased animals that have died as well as parts of animals not suitable for human consumption.

But cows are herbivores, not meat eaters, and they cannot remain healthy on a diet not designed by God for them to eat. Even cows that die from Mad Cow Disease are ground up and fed back to cows again. This insane cycle led to the recent outbreak of Mad Cow Disease in the UK, nearly wiping out the beef industry in that country. It was a tragedy waiting to happen.

Following all the modern factory farming methods, Howard Lyman turned a small family organic farm into a large corporate chemical farm and feedlot raising thousands of dairy and beef cattle, chickens, pigs and turkeys. He also grew thousands of acres of crops and employed thirty people. This was no small operation.

But Mr Lyman sold off his farm and is now a vegan. Today he is a keen advocate for vegetarianism and fights against the very cruel farming methods he once employed himself. This change in Mr Lyman came in 1979 when a spinal tumor left him paralyzed from the waist down.[31]

In 1996, Lyman appeared on the Oprah Winfrey Show at the time when mad cow disease was sparking panic worldwide. He said that one hundred thousand cows are killed every day, and that many of these cows are ground up and fed back to other cows. If only one of them has mad cow disease, warned Lyman, it had the potential to infect thousands. On the show, Lyman said…[32]

> *What we should be doing is exactly what nature says: we should have them eating grass, not other cows. We've not only turned them into carnivores, we've turned them into cannibals. [Howard Lyman]*

After hearing that cows are ground up and fed back to other cows, Winfrey said to her audience "It has just stopped me cold from eating another burger! I'm stopped!"[33] After the show, beef prices dropped to mid-1950's levels and the volume of sales also went into depression that continued for about 11 weeks. This was dubbed the Oprah Crash.[34]

Of course, ranchers and cattlemen didn't like this at all, so Texan cattle ranchers filed a suit against Lyman and Winfrey, claiming that they were "lambasting the American cattle industry" and placing "unfounded and unwarranted fear in the beef consumer's mind." And so, Lyman and Winfrey were the first Americans to defend themselves against so-called food-disparagement laws making it illegal to question the quality of food without scientific proof. These laws have been passed in some states of the US despite serious concerns regarding their constitutionality.[35]

In 1998, the state court in Texas found in favor of Lyman and Winfrey. Not to be discouraged, the case was appealed and the original verdict was upheld. Finally, after years of legal wrangling and millions of dollars spent, a Federal Judge dismissed the case. The first lawsuit testing the food disparagement laws had finally ended.[36]

Worker Abuse

Not only are animals treated with abuse, but slaughterhouse and meat packing workers are arguably engaged in one of the most dangerous factory jobs in the western world. These workers, apart from being poorly paid, endure hazardous working conditions. Any union organization or action is swiftly crushed by the companies employing them.

A 175-page report titled Blood, Sweat and Fear: Workers' Rights in US Meat and Poultry Plants, from the Human Rights Watch organization, shows how the increasing volume and speed of production coupled with close quarters, poor training and insufficient safeguards have made slaughter and boning work extremely hazardous. On a typical shift, workers can make up to 30,000 hand-cutting motions with sharp knives, causing massive repetitive motion injuries and frequent lacerations. The report has this to say about working conditions...[37]

> *Nearly every worker interviewed for this report bore physical signs of a serious injury suffered from working in a meat or poultry plant. Their accounts of life in the factories graphically explain those injuries. Automated lines carrying dead animals and their parts for disassembly move too fast for worker safety. Repeating thousands of cutting motions during each work shift puts enormous traumatic stress on workers' hands, wrists, arms, shoulders and backs. They often work in close quarters creating additional dangers for themselves and co-workers. They often receive little training and are not always given the safety equipment they need. They are often forced to work long overtime hours under pain of dismissal if they refuse. Meat and poultry industry employers set up the workplaces and practices that create these dangers, but they treat the resulting mayhem as a normal, natural part of the production process, not as what it is—repeated violations of international human rights standards. In addition to employer responsibility, however, some workplace health and safety laws and regulations fall short of international standards. [Human Rights Watch]*

One such company in North Carolina, where 5,000 workers slaughter, cut and package about 25,000 pigs per day, created an internal police force with state-sanctioned public police powers to arrest workers who were active union supporters. Many of the intimidated workers were immigrants with poor English language and communication difficulties.[38]

Live Export Shame

Live export of animals is big business for Australia, and is singled out here because the Australian live export trade is by far the largest of any country in the world. Live exports in 2002 were 970,000 head of cattle, 6.6 million sheep, 135,500 goats and 3,000 buffalo, a trade worth a total of $1.1 billion.[39]

In August 2003, the Cormo Express set sail for Saudi Arabia with a shipment of 57,937 live sheep. However, the sheep were rejected on grounds that they were diseased, leaving the Cormo Express and its live cargo in limbo for some seven weeks before another country could be found to take them. The sheep had to be purchased back from the Saudi's for $4.5 million dollars. During that time, the sheep were subjected to extremely high temperatures, with 5,581 dying of heat exhaustion and other reasons, about 9.6% of the original cargo. The sheep spent a total of eleven weeks at sea.[40]

In October 2003, the Australian Government launched a review of the live trade industry by a committee of five people, but none were represented by any animal welfare organizations, not even the RSPCA. The committee only considered the "farm to discharge into the market," that is, there was no consideration of what happens to the animals when they are unloaded at the destination port.[41]

The Australian RSPCA (Royal Society for Prevention of

Cruelty to Animals) has this to say about the live animal trade...[42]

> *These figures are a damning indictment of this cruel trade, but the actual death tolls were rarely reported at the time. Initial reports to the public often vastly underestimate the number of animals involved in such tragic incidents. In the case of the Becrux, it was 14 days before the true extent of the disaster was revealed: the death rate was five times that quoted in the original reports. And, in addition to the 880 cattle that died on the Becrux, early reports failed to mention the 1,400 sheep that also perished at sea. During July and August 2002 a further four shipments resulted in the deaths of another 14,500 sheep. [RSPCA]*

Unfortunately for the animals, profit is a greater concern than their welfare. This concern for profit even extends to the Australian Prime Minister...[43]

> *I understand the concern [regarding live trade animal cruelty] but people should bear in mind, of course, that it's a very valuable and important trade. It's worth about a billion dollars a year in export earnings and employs about 9,000 people, particularly valuable to farming in regional areas of Australia. So I deplore cruelty, any ordinary human being would and does. But we have to keep these things in perspective, we have to remember that you are talking about a very valuable economic asset and surely the goal*

*is to make the trade as humane as possible.
Isn't that the goal and that's the best thing to
do rather than ban it. [John Howard]*

The Australian Government, through the Department of Agriculture, Fisheries and Forestry state that only a 2% or more death rate will trigger a full investigation into any voyage. Death rates, however, have in fact dropped to 0.11% and 0.79% in 2003 for cattle and sheep respectively.[44]

These percentages sound inconsequential, don't they? So, let us do the arithmetic...

Cattle: 970,000 x 0.11% = 1,067
Sheep: 6,600,000 x 0.79% = 52,140

I am sure that the 1,067 cattle and the 52,140 sheep that died were not well pleased that the "mortality associated with live animal export has greatly improved as a result of Australian Government and industry action over recent years."[45]

Animal Testing

Apart from the billions of animals that suffer in factory farms, countless millions more suffer in laboratories for the sake of scientific experimentation, particularly medical experiments, as well as cosmetic and other product testing. In 1997, in the United Kingdom alone, approximately 2.64 million animal experiments involving mice, rats, guinea pigs, birds, fish, rabbits, dogs, cats and primates were carried out.[46] According to The Body Shop, the cosmetic retailer fighting against animal experimentation, the most common experiment is to drip material on rabbits' ears, or applying it to the shaved backs of rabbits and guinea pigs and studying the resulting irritation.[47]

Cosmetics, from hand creams to lipsticks to perfumes, are tested on animals for a wide range of side effects. Despite huge resistance from the cosmetic industry, the European Union has passed laws banning the use of animals for testing cosmetics, and will take effect in 2009 as a compromise deal. Britain, Germany, Austria, Belgium and the Netherlands have already banned cosmetic tests on animals.[48]

Those who advocate non-animal medical experimentation recognize that changing the status quo is difficult, but nonetheless achievable...[49]

> *The process of replacing animals in research, testing, and education is supported by studies showing that routine laboratory procedures and typical laboratory environments are more stressful for animals than is commonly appreciated. Nonetheless, the challenges of replacing animals are often considerable, raising major scientific, economic, and regulatory issues. The exploration and implementation of non-animal methods should be a priority for investigators and research institutions and should take advantage of a wide variety of viewpoints to ensure progress toward scientific, human health, and animal protection goals. [Physicians Committee for Responsible Medicine]*

Alternatives to medical animal testing include epidemiological studies (comparative studies of different human populations), computer modeling, using human cells, in-vitro research and other non-animal methods.

Deforestation

As we have seen, the global population of animals raised for food is some 20 billion livestock animals and 15.7 billion poultry birds. With the majority of these animals being raised in high-density factory farms, grain has to be grown to feed them. In 1900, only 10% of total grain grown was used to feed livestock, but this figure has grown to 45%, with the U.S. leading at 60%[50]

Deforestation is the act of clearing rainforest, old-growth forests and woodlands for domestic and commercial purposes. In 2001, it is estimated that 16.1 million hectares of tropical rainforest were cleared from the face of the earth (about 0.51 hectares every second, a good sized house block), mostly in Argentina, Brazil, Congo, Indonesia, Mexico and some African nations.[51] It is estimated that in 1900, the area of tropical rainforest was 1,093 million hectares, while today, it has been reduced to 810 million hectares.[52, 53]

> *The deforestation rate in the world's largest jungle [the Amazon] jumped 40 percent in the 12 months to the middle of 2002, and the authors of the report are bracing for figures for the subsequent year that could be yet higher. [Reuters, April 1, 2004]*

So, more and more land is being taken to satisfy our affluent western meat eating habits. The World Bank reports that cities take only 1.5 percent of earth's land, but farms occupy 36 percent. As the world population climbs towards 8.5 billion in 2040, it will become even clearer how food governs world land use. Unless we bolster our efforts to produce higher yielding crops, we face a plow-down of much of the world's remaining forests for low-yield crops and livestock.[54]

The most direct causes of deforestation are logging (both for timber and paper manufacture), agriculture, cattle grazing, mining and oil exploration. Notice that this list does not include human population growth, which is actually an insignificant cause of deforestation. Forests have been converted for cattle in Central America, soybean production in Brazil to provide animal feed, and pulpwood in Indonesia. One of the main drivers of deforestation is the huge US fast food and hamburger market, with its demand for low-quality cheap meat, while intensive meat production in Europe requires ever-increasing feed for livestock.[55]

The large-scale destruction of tropical rain forests and consequent loss of rich, complex ecosystems is one of the most globally important environmental issues today, and a number of serious consequences occur as a result. These include...

Greenhouse Gasses: Forests act as the lungs of the earth by absorbing carbon dioxide from the atmosphere and replacing it with oxygen. When forests are cleared, the trees are mostly burnt or left to decay (this is the case even for logging, where only the trunks are taken out of the forest, with branches and foliage left behind). This leads to an increase in carbon dioxide and reduction in oxygenation of the atmosphere. Some 35% of carbon dioxide now found in the atmosphere is due to deforestation and conversion of prairie, woodlands and forested ecosystems into agricultural systems as well as causing increases in methane and nitrous oxide.[56]

Soil Erosion, Silting and Flooding: Deforestation causes a multitude of effects such as degradation of soil quality, loss of shade, soil erosion and drying out of the base soil. Rain falling in cleared forest areas is not absorbed by the soil or vegetation, but instead runs off the denuded ground. Heavy rainfall dramatically increases surface run off and soil erosion. Serious flooding results from the huge volumes of water that was once absorbed by the lush vegetation. Significant silting then occurs in rivers, lakes and dams due to the increased soil being carried by the waters. Soil fertility decreases by 80% in only just a few years after forest removal.[57]

Extinction: Although tropical forests cover only about 10% of earth's land surface, they still contain about half of all of the world's flora and fauna species. Rainforests harbor about one third of the total number of birds, mammals and amphibians. Even in a single acre, hundreds of plant and animals species can be found. Unfortunately, through deforestation, many of these animal and plant species are lost daily.[58]

Indeed, if every person on the earth ate a plant-based diet like the Genesis Diet given to us by God, there is no reason why the earth could not sustain a population of 20 billion people.

Resource Usage

As we have seen, animal grazing is a very poor utilization of available land, and calorie for calorie, is a very inefficient use of this resource. There are certainly not enough natural resources to provide an animal based diet for future population growth. This will only serve to force more and more animals into dreadfully cruel factory farms.

Industries that support today's western meat-based diet are woefully inefficient operations, and pay little regard to the environmental impact they are causing. Factory farms and associated feed crops use huge amounts of energy. This energy is obtained principally from fossil fuels used to drive machinery that harvest, transport and process grain feed, as well as running, heating and cooling the factory farms themselves. Further energy must then be expended to kill, process, transport and store the meat, organs, hides and hair obtained from the animals.

John Robbins, founder of EarthSave International, wrote this tongue-in-cheek anecdote…[59]

> *Even driving many gas-guzzling luxury cars can conserve energy over walking — that is, when the calories you burn walking come from the standard American diet! This is because the energy needed to produce the food you would burn in walking a given distance is greater than the energy needed to fuel your car to travel the same distance.*
> *[John Robbins]*

Raising animals for food and their milk also consumes huge amounts of water. A kilogram of meat requires an estimated 100,000 liters of water, about 100 times more than one kilogram of potatoes.[60] Factory farms are a huge user of water.

The Ogallala Aquifer is a huge underground reserve of water stretching over 8 states of the United States. Since the mid 1900's, use of the aquifer for its water has steadily increased, with water extraction rates now outstripping natural replenishment. A 16,000 hog-per-day slaughter house proposed for construction in Texas requested a public subsidy to use a staggering 1000 million liters per day from the aquifer for its operations.[61]

With factory farming becoming more prevalent in developing countries, where water conservation laws and infrastructure are not developed, excess water usage by the meat and livestock industry can be a catalyst for trouble. Even now, the demand for water is a serious source of friction for nations that share rivers, lakes and aquifers. United Nations figures indicate that there are some 300 potential conflicts around the world arising from squabbles over river borders and drawing water from shared lakes and aquifers.[62]

Pollution

Animals in factory farms are crowded into small areas, far smaller than they would ever use if they were allowed to live naturally. This high concentration and sheer number of animals brings about significant problems concerning the vast amount of waste produced and the methods used to dispose of it. In industrialized nations, this waste exceeds that of the human population by many times.

To compound the problems with so much manure and urine, the waste does not have to be treated like human sewerage. Instead, the waste is funneled into huge open-air lagoons the size of several football fields, where it can sit for indeterminate periods of time. Often, it is sprayed untreated onto surrounding fields.[63]

These lagoons are subject to leakage or overflow, particularly in times of heavy rains, sending dangerous microbes, bacteria, nitrates and other pollutants into fresh water streams and other water supplies. These pollutants often kill enormous amounts of fish and find their way into human drinking water, necessitating filtering and chemical treatment of the water to make it fit for consumption.[64]

High levels of nitrates in drinking water increase the risk of methemoglobinemia, or blue-baby syndrome, which can kill infants. Animal wastes also contain disease-forming pathogens, such as salmonella, E-coli, cryptosporidium, and fecal coliform. In 2000, six people, including a 2 year old gird, died in Walkerton, Ontario as a result of drinking E-coli contaminated water caused by cattle manure runoff.[65] In 1993, some 100 people died and more than 430,000 became ill when manure from dairy cows caused cryptosporidium contamination of Milwaukee's drinking water.[66]

Often, there are minimal and ineffective laws and regulations governing the odor and pollution factory farms produce. A report in the Pittsburg Post-Gazette stated that...[67]

Large factory farms are pigging out in Pennsylvania, generating huge piles of manure that threaten to degrade soil, streams and ground water, cause human health problems and pollute the air with pungent odors, according to a study by Citizens for Pennsylvania's Future. [Citizens for Pennsylvania's Future] said no state regulations control odors, air pollution and the excessive levels of phosphorus from manure that is spread on farm fields. Phosphorous and nitrogen are present in manure and other fertilizers. Both can run off farm fields and pollute local waterways and regional water bodies like the Chesapeake Bay. [Pittsburg Post-Gazette]

Excessive pollution of water with phosphorous and nitrogen from animal wastes provides the conditions for enormous bursts of algae bloom. The Dead Zone in the Gulf of Mexico is located just out from the mouth of the Mississippi River. Covering an area of some 18,000 square kilometers, there is simply not enough oxygen in the water to support aquatic life. With nearly 50% of continental United States draining its waters into the Mississippi River, including great rives such as the Missouri, Ohio, Arkansas and Red Rivers, algae bloom caused by animal wastes is a significant contributor to the dead zone.[68]

But not only is water adversely polluted, the atmosphere is polluted by factory farms, too. As the waste is decomposing in the lagoons, hundreds of volatile gasses such as nitrogen, hydrogen sulfide (rotten egg gas), ammonia and methane are released. Staggering amounts of contaminants are also released from factory farms into the atmosphere.[69]

The stench from factory farm gasses can be unbearable.

Residents living near factory farms often report disgusting odors that get so bad at times they have to leave the area. Worse still, the gasses given off not only significantly contribute to greenhouse gas emissions, they contain harmful chemicals, causing sore air passages, headaches, skin rashes, seizures and even comas.

Eric Schlosser describes such a place in the US...[70]

> *You can smell Greeley, Colorado, long before you can see it. The smell is hard to forget but not easy to describe, a combination of live animals, manure, and dead animals being rendered into dog food. The smell is worst during the summer months, blanketing Greeley day and night like an invisible fog. Many people who live there no longer notice the smell; it recedes into the background, present but not present, like the sound of traffic for New Yorkers. Other's can't stop thinking about the smell, even after years; it permeates everything, gives them headaches, makes them nauseous, interferes with their sleep. Greeley is a modern-day factory town where cattle are the main units of production, where workers and machines turn large steer into small, vacuum-sealed packages of meat. [Eric Schlosser]*

Animal Gasses

It has been estimated that, globally, livestock animals release approximately 60 million tons of methane gas annually in belches and flatulence. A single cow produces about 400 liters of methane and 1,500 liters of carbon dioxide per day.[71] All this gas is a serious problem...[72]

> *While emissions from power plants, auto tailpipes and forest fires have long been blamed for warming the planet, the innards of livestock, including sheep and goats, are now being recognized as significant contributors as well. "I know it sounds crazy, but it's a serious topic," said Ralph Cicerone, an atmospheric scientist and chancellor at the University of California, Irvine. "Methane is the second-most-important greenhouse gas in the atmosphere now. The population of beef cattle and dairy cattle has grown so much that methane from cows now is big. This is not a trivial issue." [Los Angeles Times]*

In developed countries, the proportion of methane emission from animals can be up to 50% of total emission. For example, in the UK, methane emissions from animal flatulence and belching is about 25%, while New Zealand has a staggering 90%[73]

In line with the Kyoto greenhouse gas reduction targets, New Zealand and other developed nations, have agreed to reduce their greenhouse gas emission to 1990 levels by 2012. To meet these Kyoto targets, the New Zealand government has proposed a flatulence tax on farmers of sheep, cows, deer and goats.[74]

So huge is the problem, that many scientists are busy trying to find methods to reduce the amount of methane gas produced by livestock animals. Feedlots and pastures are becoming laboratories for researchers testing all sorts of remedies, including vaccines, formulated feed, selective breeding and even bioengineering.

So, once again, the solution is to inject animals with all sorts of chemical concoctions, to dig deep into their DNA, or even add dangerous chemicals to their feed, such as chlorinated hydrocarbons found in solvents and petroleum fuels.

These scientists are even trying to replace the weight of methane in cattle with additional weight in meat or milk…[75]

> *There are plenty of reasons to keep the cows from giving off methane. It makes more sense to have it as weight on the cattle. If we can succeed, cows produce less methane and have more meat or milk. [Sherwood Rowland]*

Chemical Onslaught

Heavy metals are added to livestock feed. For example, zinc and copper are added to hog and poultry feed to prevent disease and aid digestion. Cadmium and selenium are also used and have been found to promote growth in low doses. Unfortunately, animals can only absorb so much of the metals they ingest, so the majority of these are excreted in the manure and urine. Water run-off finding its way into water storages and surrounding soils begin to build up concentrations of these metals. Heavy metal pollution is almost impossible to reverse.[76]

Fat soluble pesticides and other chemicals become concentrated in the fatty flesh of animals, ensuring a plentiful supply of poison for meat eaters. Dioxin (a component of Agent Orange), heptachlor, PCB's, toxaphene and others are very toxic.

But not only is the flesh of animals contaminated when the animal is alive, but the chemical onslaught continues after slaughter. In fact, animal flesh turns a sickly green color very quickly, and so the meat industry hides this by adding nitrates and other preservative chemicals to keep the meat looking blood red. Further chemicals are added to processed meats such as hams, bacons, sausages and the like.

The late Dr William Lijinsky was a leading toxicologist and carcinogenesis researcher, publishing over 600 research articles.[77] He discovered as early as 1963 that polycyclic aromatic hydrocarbons (PAH) carcinogens are formed in charcoaled and fried meats. He testified to the US Congress about the dangers of nitrates in preserved meats as a source of cancer in both animals and humans.

Not only do farm animals suffer from this chemical onslaught. Native animals suffer, too.

In Tasmania, the most heavily forested state of Australia, a helicopter spraying a plantation with pesticides crashed, spilling its load. Soon, after a heavy period of rain, the poisonous pesticide found its way into waters near the town of St Helens, poisoning over 90% of its oysters in January 2004.[78] Scores of people also visited their local doctors with unexplained illnesses.

Chemicals such as atrazine, simazine and sodium mono-fluoroacetate are used specifically by the logging industry to target plants, insects and native browsing animals that might slow down the rate of tree growth. These chemicals harm and kill many other animals such as Tasmanian devils, wombats, birds, crayfish and oysters.[79]

Chapter 6
BIBLICAL HEALING

God Our Redeemer and Healer

God reveals Himself under many different names, reflecting His power, redemptive nature and character. These attributes of God meet all our needs here on earth.

Elohim: This is the name given to God in the very first verse of the Bible "In the beginning, God (Elohim) created the heavens and the earth" (Genesis 1:1). The *im* ending denotes plurality, reflecting the triune nature of God — Father, Son and Holy Spirit. In the Old Testament, the name Elohim designates might and power.

El-Shaddai: The Hebrew meaning of the word Shaddai is translated "breast" thus the name El-Shaddai denotes one who nourishes, supplies and comforts — one who pours out blessings to His people.

> **By the God [El] of your father who will help you, and by the Almighty [Shaddai] who will bless you with blessings of heaven above, blessings of the deep that lies beneath, blessings of the breasts and of the womb. Genesis 49:25**

Adonai: This name for God denotes ownership. As we accept Jesus as our Lord and Savior, it is no longer we that live, but Christ that lives within us (Galatians 2:20). We have been redeemed by the blood of Jesus and therefore sons of the living God, requiring our obedience and submission to Him (1 Thessalonians 1:8).

Jehovah: This name for God is derived from the Hebrew "Yahweh" simply meaning "I Am". When Moses asked in who's name he was being sent to Egypt, God simply replied, "I AM WHO I AM" (Exodus 3:14).

Jehovah Shammah: The Lord is present. This name for God is found in the last verse of Ezekiel (Ezekiel 48:35), who wrote about Judah's future restoration after the fall of Jerusalem. The city would be given a new name, meaning "The Lord is There."

Jehovah M'Kaddesh: The Lord is our sanctifier (Leviticus 20:8). The term sanctify means "to set apart" indicating that we should be setting ourselves apart from the world and not partake in its evil practices. A good example is 1 Thessalonians 4:3 where Paul exhorts Christians to abstain from sexual immorality.

Jehovah Shalom: The Lord is our peace (Judges 6:24). This name for God reflects the nature of Jesus, the Prince of Peace (Isaiah 9:6). Being justified through faith, we have peace with God through Jesus Christ our Lord (Romans 5:1).

Jehovah Rohi: The Lord is our shepherd (Psalm 23:1). This name essentially means "lead to pasture", as a shepherd would lead his flock. Jesus described himself as the Good Shepherd, who knows His sheep (John 10:14).

Jehovah Jireh: The Lord is our provider (Genesis 22:8). This name for God is set within the narrative of Abraham being required to sacrifice his son Isaac as a burnt offering. When Isaac queried Abraham the whereabouts of the lamb to be sacrificed, Abraham replied that God would provide.

Jehovah Nissi: The Lord is our banner (Exodus 17:15). This name was given to God after Israel's victory over the Amalekites, when an alter was erected as a sign of deliverance and salvation from the enemy. In the book of Isaiah, God's people were urged to lift up a banner on the high mountain when the Lord of hosts mustered His army for battle (Isaiah 13:2).

Jehovah Tsidkenu: The Lord is our righteousness (Jeremiah 23:6). This name for God appears in Jeremiah's prophecy of a "Branch of Righteousness" and a "King" who will appear, namely, Jesus, to whom it was "accounted to him for righteousness" (Romans 4:22).

Jehovah Rapha: The Lord is our healer (Exodus 15:26). God is a healer — it is His nature. He wants to heal and free His people from all manner of disease, affliction and emotional trauma.

> **If you diligently heed the voice of the Lord your God and do what is right in His sight, give ear to His commandments and keep His statutes, I will put none of these diseases on you which I have brought on the Egyptians. For I am the Lord who heals you. Exodus 15:26**

Jesus died on the cross for our sins, that is certain, and many Christians understand the redemptive nature of His life and death. What is not always fully recognized, however, is that Jesus also suffered and died for our infirmities and sicknesses. He is clearly both Savior *and* Healer. Our attitude to healing should be the same as our attitude to forgiveness; both have been dealt with once and for all.

> **But He was wounded for our transgressions, He was bruised for our iniquities; the chastisement for our peace was upon Him, and by His stripes we are healed. Isaiah 53:5**

When evening had come, they brought to Him many who were demon-possessed. And He cast out the spirits with a word, and healed all who were sick, that it might be fulfilled which was spoken by Isaiah the prophet, saying: "He Himself took our infirmities and bore our sicknesses". Matthew 8:16-17

Salvation and healing are therefore twin redemptive blessings that Jesus brought to the world. There is salvation for the spirit, and healing of the body, perfect deliverance of our entire being.

For you were bought at a price; therefore glorify God in your body and in your spirit, which are God's. 1 Corinthians 6:20

The last supper reflects the dual nature of Jesus' purpose; the wine representing Jesus shedding His blood for our sins, and the bread representing His body that was broken for us. This is the same body that was lacerated with stripes for our healing, and bruised for our iniquities, the body that has taken our infirmities and has borne our sicknesses. Both sin and sickness continue to lose their power as we grow and believe in faith the work Jesus has done for us.

Jesus healed wherever he went, with the Gospels giving numerous examples of his healing grace to all those who sought Him, never turning anybody away. Some examples of healing in the Gospel of Matthew include lepers (Matthew 8:3), Peter's mother-in-law (Matthew 8:15), multitudes (Matthew 4:23, 8:16, 9:15, 9:33, 14:36, 15:30, 17:18, 19:2), demon possession (Matthew 8:32, 9:33, 12:22), paralytics (Matthew 9:6), issues of blood (Matthew 9:22), and blindness (Matthew 9:30, 20:34). Jesus even gave His disciples authority to do the same (Matthew 10:1), and this authority has not been revoked today.

And these signs will follow those who believe:

In my name they will cast out demons; they will speak with new tongues; they will take up serpents; and if they drink anything deadly; it will by no means hurt them; they will lay hands on the sick, and they will recover. Mark 16:17-18

The disciples continued to minister healing. In the book of Acts, we see healing miracles in the name of Jesus, such as healing of paralytics (Acts 3:6-7, 8:7, 9:34, 14:10), demonic deliverance (Acts 8:7, 16:18, 19:12), resurrections from the dead (Acts 9:40, 20:10), signs and wonders (Acts 14:3), and fever (Acts 28:8).

The Word of God is supernatural medicine, working through our spirit to touch our physical bodies.

Faith that God Has Healed

Faith is what drives the Christian to believe in the Word of God and promises of God. It is a projection of the mind's eye towards those things that God has already promised us. In the great faith chapter of Hebrews (chapter 11), faith is described as the surety of things hoped for and the certainty of the things we cannot see (Hebrews 11:1). Hope is important, of course, but it only receives substance when it is driven by faith.

It is by faith that many of old were drawn to do extraordinary things...

By faith we know that God formed the universe by His word (Hebrews 11:3)

By faith Abel offered a more excellent sacrifice than Cain (Hebrews 11:4)

By faith Enoch was translated and did not see death (Hebrews 11:5)

By faith Noah prepared an ark for the saving of his household (Hebrews 11:7)

By faith Abraham obeyed when called to live in the Promised Land (Hebrews 11:9)

By faith Sarah conceived a child well past child bearing age (Hebrews 11:11)

By faith Abraham offered Isaac as a sacrifice (Hebrews 11:17)

By faith Isaac blessed Jacob and Esau (Hebrews 11:20)

By faith Jacob blessed each of the sons of Joseph (Hebrews 11:21)

By faith Joseph mentioned the departure of the children of Israel (Hebrews 11:22)

By faith Moses was hidden in the reeds (Hebrews 11:23)

By faith Moses refused to be called the son of Pharaoh (Hebrews 11:24)

By faith Moses departed from Egypt, not fearing the wrath of Pharaoh (Hebrews 11:27)

By faith Moses kept the Passover so that the first-born of Israel would be safe (Hebrews 11:28).

By faith the children of Israel passed through the Red Sea (Hebrews 11:29)

By faith the walls of Jericho fell after being encircled seven days (Hebrews 11:30)

By faith Rahab received spies in her house (Hebrews 11:31)

By faith Gideon, Barak, Samson, Jepthah, David, Samuel and the prophets conquered kingdoms and performed many other mighty works (Hebrews 11:32-34)

In our own lives and circumstances, we can believe God in faith that He will heal sick and infirm people, that he will save those who may seem to be beyond saving (indeed, nobody in this world is beyond saving), and that He will deliver on all His promises.

> **Without faith it is impossible to please Him, for he who comes to God must believe that He is, and that He is a rewarder of those who seek Him. Hebrews 11:6**

Faith is very powerful. It can move "mountains" in our lives. What greater mountain removal is there than deliverance from some disease or affliction?

> **If you have faith as a mustard seed, you can say to this mulberry tree, 'Be pulled up by the roots and be planted in the sea,' and it would obey you. Luke 17:6**

It is God's will for us to be healthy and well. Acting on that promise through faith will ensure that we can live a healthy life free of disease and infirmities until He takes away our breath and returns us to dust (Psalm 104:29).

When I returned from hospital after being diagnosed with diabetes, I began to study what God's word had to say about health, healing and diet. As I read, more faith began to swell up in me. I remember saying to my wife, "This is only temporary, and God has healed me." Within four months, I was off insulin and medication, and within a further 12 months or so, I had lost over 30 kilograms in weight. I have never felt better for a long time.

> **Then your light shall break forth like the morning, your healing shall spring forth speedily, and your righteousness shall go before you; the glory of he Lord shall be your guard. Isaiah 58:8**

This book is a result of that faith in God that he has healed me, my wife and my family. We continue to believe in God for continued healing and maintenance of good health. We believe, in faith, that God will keep us well even into our senior years. From Genesis to Revelation, there are two themes: the will of God to free us from sin and its penalty, and to heal us from all our infirmities and diseases. Faith is a decisive act of trust in Him.

Consider the healing of the epileptic boy in Matthew chapter 17. The boy's father approached Jesus asking for mercy for his son, reporting that the disciples could not heal him. Jesus replied with a rebuke, "How long will I stay with you? How long will I put up with you?" After rebuking the demon and healing the boy, Jesus' disciples enquired why they could not drive out the demon. To this, Jesus replied, "Because you have so little faith." (Matthew 17:20).

It should be clear that God's will is to heal. This needs to be affirmed by each one of us who believes. It is not a question of whether God *may* heal us, but faith in the knowledge that He has *already* healed us.

Name of Jesus

As believers in Jesus, we can ask God for healing and

receive it. This power of healing comes from invoking the name of Jesus Christ, so we can confidently use this name because He has conquered sin and death. It is the name above all other names (Philippians 2:9).

> **Most assuredly, I say to you, whatever you ask the Father in my name He will give to you. John 16:24**

This power in Jesus' name is still active today just as it was at the time of His ministry on earth and the Acts of the Apostles.

> **Then Peter said, "Silver and gold I do not have, but what I have I give to you: In the name of Jesus Christ of Nazareth, rise up and walk." Acts 3:6**

As believers in Jesus, we can ask God for healing in His name and know that we will receive it.

Anointing With Oil

The book of James gives specific instruction for those who are sick to call upon the elders of the church, who are to pray in faith in the name of Jesus and anoint them with oil.

> **Is anyone among you sick? Let him call for the elders of the church, and let them pray over him, anointing him with oil in the name of the Lord. And the prayer of faith will save the sick, and the Lord will raise him up. And if he has committed sins, he will be forgiven. James 5:14-15**

Thus the prayer of faith will both deliver from sickness and provide forgiveness of sin.

Laying Of Hands

Believers can lay hands on the sick, and in faith, believe that the sick will recover. Corporate laying on of hands by a group of Christians is a very powerful healing weapon, when the whole group affirms that by His stripes the sick person has been healed.

> **They will lay hands on the sick, and they will recover. Mark 16:18**

> **And it happened that the father of Publius lay sick of a fever and dysentery. Paul went in to him and prayed, and he laid his hands on him and he healed him. Acts 28:8**

Losing Our Healing

Is it possible to lose our healing? Indeed, it is, and it can happen subtly over time or quickly as an attack. This comes about by a number of factors.

Doubt

The first and foremost method of losing healing is losing faith, or doubting what God has provided for us. Continued positive confession that He has borne our griefs and carried our sorrows, that He was wounded for our transgressions and by His stripes we are healed ensures any modicum of doubt will be quashed.

God's word in our hearts that finds expression in what we say is very powerful. So too is negative confession. When seeds of doubt enter our minds, we can speak words of death regarding our healing. We must always confess that Jesus has already paid the price for our healing.

Unconfessed Sin

Weakness and sickness can come upon believers when

they harbor unconfessed sin. Sickness due to unconfessed sin is remedied by confessing that sin, repenting of it, and turning away from it.

> **For this reason many are weak and sick among you, and many sleep. For if we would judge ourselves, we would not be judged. But when we are judged, we are chastened by the Lord, that we may not be condemned with the world. 1 Corinthians 11:30-32**

Demonic Attack

Satan is the cunning serpent (Genesis 3:1), inflictor of disease (Job 2;7), opposer (Zechariah 3:1), tempter (Matthew 4:3), ruler of demons (Matthew 12:24), wicked one (Matthew 13:19), claimer of false authority (Luke 4:6), murderer, liar and father of lies (John 8:44), prompter of sin (John 13:2), ruler of this world (John 14:30), power of darkness (Acts 26:18), blinder of minds of unbelievers (2 Corinthians 4:4), corruptor of minds (2 Corinthians 11:3), prince of the power of the air (Ephesians 2:2), contender of the saints (Ephesians 6:12), author of lying wonders (2 Thessalonians 2:9), seeker of whom he may devour (1 Peter 5:8), accuser of the brethren (Revelation 12:10) and the dragon and serpent of old (Revelation 20:2). He is one bad dude, but remember that Jesus has defeated him, and Jesus now holds the keys to Hades and Death (Revelation 1:18).

Demons are spirits in the Satanic hierarchy that do not have bodies and they long to possess one in order to express themselves and inflict harm to the person being possessed. If they can't find a human, then sometimes animals will do (Matthew 8:31). Demons seek to enter humans wherever and whenever they can, and they will never rest until they find possession.

Just as God uses human instruments to encourage and bless others by the power of the Holy Spirit, demons use vulnerable people to destroy each other. One such method of destruction is to bring about sickness and disease.

Now when the sun was setting, all those who had anyone sick with various diseases brought them to Him; and He laid His hands on every one of them and healed them. And demons also came out, crying out and saying, "You are the Christ, the Son of God!" And He, rebuking them, did not allow them to speak, for they knew He was the Christ. Luke 4:40-41

And Jesus rebuked the demon, and he came out of him [the epileptic]; and the child was cured from that very hour. Matthew 17:18

Unhealthy Living

Unfortunately, attention to diet, exercise and lifestyle are not generally covered in otherwise excellent Christian books concerning healing. This book is one attempt to address this imbalance.

Healthy living and proper diet are vital in keeping sickness at bay. It must be remembered that we live in a realm of natural laws of physics, chemistry and biology — laws that God Himself established when He created the heavens and the earth.

Therefore, it is possible to receive healing and be made whole, only to fritter that healing away with a life-time of poor diet, lack of exercise, or vices such as smoking and drinking alcohol to excess. There can be no doubt that much of the sickness and disease in today's modern world, even among Christians who have been healed by His stripes, are due to poor eating habits.

Unscriptual Teaching on Healing

As we have already seen, Jesus bore our sins and our diseases on the cross. When we believed in Jesus as our Lord and Savior, and confessed our sins to Him, we have His guarantee that we are saved. Similarly, the moment that we believe and confess that Jesus bore our infirmities and sicknesses, that is the moment we are healed.

This means that sickness has no business in the Christian's life, but unfortunately, sometimes we are taught that God is the author of sickness because he either wants us to suffer, or because he needs to punish us. This could not be further from the truth.

Chastisement

Some say that God brings on sickness as a form of chastisement, or punishment for a wrong-doing. This idea comes from the following verse...

> **My son, do not despise the chastening of the Lord, nor detest His correction; For whom the Lord loves He corrects, just as a father the son in whom he delights. Proverbs 3:11-12**

Now, what earthly father would want to punish his children by inflicting them with cancer or heart disease? The scripture does not say God will impart a disease to teach us a lesson, but rather, the dictionary definition of the word "chastening" means to punish or discipline, to restrain and moderate, or to purify. None of these mean that God will smite us with some sort of disease that will one day kill us. The meaning of this verse is therefore one of correction. It is akin to parents disciplining their child to correct his ways.

Suffering

Suffering for Jesus does not mean that we should

contract some disease. This false teaching comes from the following verse…

But may the God of all grace, who called us to His eternal glory by Christ Jesus, after you have suffered for a while, perfect, establish, strengthen and settle you. 1 Peter 5:10

The suffering referred to in this verse is the disappointments, hardships, persecutions, tumults, trials and temptations that can often come by in a Christian's life. God promises us a victorious life, not one free of all problems.

Consider the apostles, who were imprisoned, beaten, mocked and persecuted. They simply…

…departed from the presence of the council, rejoicing that they were counted worthy to suffer shame for His name. Acts 5:41

Indeed, there is blessing in suffering for Jesus' sake, and we can even rejoice that the Lord has counted us worthy.

But even if you should suffer for righteousness' sake, you are blessed. "And do not be afraid of their threats, nor be troubled." 1 Peter 3:14

Like chastisement, it may not be comfortable at the time, but there is divine purpose, for "we know that all things work together for good to those who love God, to those who are called according to His purpose" (Romans 8:28).

Afflictions

Like sufferings, the righteous in God can expect to receive afflictions, meaning trials, persecutions and temptations.

Many are the afflictions of the righteous, but

the Lord delivers him out of them all. Psalm 34:19

Again, the word "affliction" does not denote sickness, disease or physical disablement. How can God be glorified in His people if He wills that they be inflicted with all manner of diseases? Thus, through trials and temptations, we must all allow ourselves to grow in our walk with Him, and the promise is that He will deliver us from them all!

Paul's Thorn in the Flesh

One objection to spiritual healing is Paul's "thorn in the flesh". This is the idea that God inflicted upon Paul some sort of disease in order to keep him on the straight and narrow.

And lest I should be exalted above measure by the abundance of revelations, a thorn in the flesh was given to me, a messenger from Satan to buffet me, lest I be exalted above measure. Concerning this thing I pleaded with the Lord three times that it might depart from me. And He said to me, "My grace is sufficient for you, for My strength is made perfect in weakness." 2 Corinthians 12:7-8

Paul's thorn was not a disease, as Paul himself states that it was a "messenger from Satan to buffet" him. The word "buffet" means to toss from side to side, like a boat in a storm being buffeted in the waves. This is confirmation that Satan's attempt to thwart us increases as our faith in God increases. Paul was opposed, mobbed, expelled, beaten, jailed, disputed against, tried in court, whipped, beaten with rods, stoned, shipwrecked, in perils from water, robbers and heathens, hungry and thirsty, cold and naked, amongst other things (2 Corinthians 11:24-28). In this list, disease or sickness has not once been mentioned. The Bible says nothing of Paul ever being sick or having some disease.

The purpose of Paul's thorn in the flesh was to stop him

from becoming self-exalted through the numerous revelations he was receiving from the Lord. Furthermore, Paul's thorn in the flesh never incapacitated his ability to perform his ministry.

CONCLUSION

A s outlined in this book, there is no doubt that the healthiest possible diet is vegetarian, in particular, the plant-only based Genesis diet described in the first book of the Bible. In Genesis 1:29 and 30, we see that God gave all manner of fruits and herbs (vegetables and other plant foods) to eat, both for man and animals.

> **And God said, See, I have given you every herb that yields seed which is on the face of the earth, and every tree whose fruit yields seed; to you it shall be for food. And it was so. Genesis 1:29**

Dr Henry Morris, president of the Institute of Creation Research, explains it like this…[1]

> *It was not intended that either man or animals should eat animal food. As far as carnivorous animals are concerned, this must also have been a later development, either at the time of the Curse or after the Flood. Even today, such animals can (and do) live on a vegetarian diet. [Dr Henry M. Morris]*

Without Genesis 1:29 as a key verse, it would be very difficult to mount a case for vegetarianism in Christian circles, other than to argue on the grounds of health, environmental care and animal welfare (which in themselves are still strong arguments).

But even with Genesis 1:29, there are numerous references to eating animal foods in the Bible, and actually only just a few references to vegetarianism. Indeed, directly after the Flood, God specifically allowed the eating of animal flesh...

Every moving thing that lives shall be food for you. I have given you all things, even as the green herbs. Genesis 9:3

So why is there this apparent dilemma? Here, God allows the eating of animals (albeit with the proviso that the meat should not be eaten with the blood). If the Genesis diet originated from God, and God only wants what is good for us, why then did he allow us to eat animal flesh?

There is no easy answer to this. Those who advocate vegetarian diets, like in this book, point to Genesis 1:29, and those who eat meat point to Genesis 9:3. Indeed, the eating of meat is not condemned in the Bible, nor is vegetarianism specifically promoted.

Some have argued that Jesus Himself was a vegetarian. However, this cannot be the case, as the Bible records on two occasions that he ate flesh: once in Luke chapter 22 where he desired to eat the Passover meal (which includes the eating of lamb - see Exodus 12:8), and the other in Luke 24:42-43 when, after His resurrection, He ate bread and fish. Moreover, Jesus himself did not condemn the eating of animal flesh, as is evidenced by the fact that He blessed the fish that fed five thousand (Matthew 14:19). He even assisted Simon to catch a whole boatload of fish (Luke 5:4).

In the Gospels and Epistles, there is no specific reference to the type of diet that Jesus followed. Indeed, the only direct reference to what Jesus ate (or at least, would eat) is found in the great Immanuel Prophecy of Isaiah chapter 7. Here we see that Jesus was to eat curds and honey (Isaiah 7:15). All that can really be said of Jesus is that he would have eaten a diet high in fruits, vegetables, legumes and grains that was typically eaten in Mediterranean and Middle Eastern countries at that time. Meat was only eaten on special occasions, such as in the Passover feast.

Jesus shed his own blood and has borne the sin of all mankind onto Himself. Therefore, the need to shed innocent animal blood for atonement as required by the Old Testament Jews now no longer applies. Although we are allowed to eat animal flesh, there is no compelling reason to do so today, particularly in our modern world with its abundance of available produce and modern transport logistics. There is no longer any need to kill animals for survival that may have been required by our pioneers.

To eat meat or not to eat meat is not a new issue, even in the Church. At the time of Paul the Apostle, the eating of meat was a hot topic, of which he said this…

Let not him who eats despise him who does not eat, and let not him who does not eat judge him who eats, for God has received him. Romans 14:3

Therefore do not let your good be spoken of as evil, for the kingdom of God is not food and drink, but righteousness and peace and joy in the Holy Spirit. For he who serves Christ in these things is acceptable to God and approved by man. Therefore let us pursue the things which make for peace and the things that by which one may edify another. Do not destroy the works of God for the sake of food. All things indeed are pure, but it is evil for the man who eats with offence. Romans 14:16-20

Clearly, for the sake of righteousness, peace and joy in the Spirit, vegetarians must not judge meat-eaters, and meat-eaters must not judge vegetarians. This is particularly true of vegetarians, who can at times become puffed up with pride and self-righteousness, even if for the best of intentions. From the point of view of salvation, it makes no difference whether one eats flesh or not. To eat meat is therefore not a sin, but to eat too much of it, like we do in western society, has a most deleterious effect on our health.

Thus, the decision to be a vegetarian cannot be a religious one, at least not in Christianity. Rather, the decision is personal, and many come to that decision via different paths. Some choose because they want to restore health, some because they abhor cruelty to animals, and some because they are concerned about the environment. Whatever the reason, Christianity can, and should, embrace vegetarianism for the reasons outlined in this book.

Now all this does not mean that meat-eaters should ignore vegetarian arguments. The majority of vegetarians, including many Christians, are converts from meat eating, rather than from a vegetarian upbringing.

It has been proven over and over again a diet rich in fruits and vegetables promotes better health, staves off many of today's lifestyle diseases such as cancer, heart disease, stroke and diabetes, and increases longevity and quality of life. Indeed, the choice of food can often be a choice of life, or a choice of death.

I call heaven and earth as witnesses today against you, that I have set before you life and death, blessing and cursing, therefore, choose life, that both you and your descendents may live. Deuteronomy 30:19

May God bless you and keep you well!

APPENDIX A
FURTHER READING

Books

Archer, John, On the Water Front, ISBN 0646043188

Attwood, Dr Charles (MD), Dr Attwood's Low Fat Prescription for Kids, ISBN 0670858293

Barnard, Dr Neal (MD), Food for Life, ISBN 0517882019

Barnard, Dr Neal (MD), Turn off the Fat Genes, ISBN 073291096X

Barnard, Dr Neal (MD), Eat Right, Live Longer, ISBN 05178877889

Barnard, Dr Neal (MD), Foods the Fight Pain, ISBN 0553812378

Barnard, Dr Neal (MD), Foods That Cause You to Lose Weight, ISBN 0553812378

Banik, Dr Allen (MD), The Choice is Clear, ISBN 0911311319

Batmanghelidj, F. (MD), Your Body's Many Cries for Water, ISBN 0962994235

Bragg, Paul C., The Miracle of Fasting, ISBN 0877900361

Bragg, Paul C., Water. The Shocking Truth, ISBN 0877900639

Bragg, Paul C., Apple Cider Vinegar, ISBN 0877900442

Cherry, Reginald (MD), The Bible Cure, ISBN 088419535X

Cohen, Jay (MD), Over Dose, The Case Against the Drug Companies, ISBN 1585421235

Colbert, Don (MD), Toxic Relief, ISBN 0884197603

Gaynor, Mitchel (MD), Cancer Prevention Program, ISBN 1575663821

Hughes, Rebecca, Walking for Health and Fitness, ISBN 0881764965

Jackson & Soothill, Is the Medicine Making You Ill? ISBN 0207157960

Jensen, Bernard (DC), Tissue Cleaning Through Bowel Management, ISBN 0895295849

Lau, Benjamin (MD), Garlic For Health, ISBN 0941524329

Malkmus, George, Why Christians Get Sick, ISBN 1560438495

McDougall, John (MD), The McDougall Program for a Healthy Heart, ISBN 0525938680

Mindell, Earl, Garlic, The Miracle Nutrient, ISBN 0879836490

Ornish, Dr Dean (MD), Dr Dean Ornish's Program for Reversing Heart Disease, ISBN 0804110387

Robbins, John, Diet for A New America, ISBN 0915811812

Robbins, John, The Food Revolution, ISBN 1573247022

Physicians Committee for Responsible Medicine, Healthy Eating for Life to Prevent and Treat Diabetes, ISBN 0471435988

Physicians Committee for Responsible Medicine, Healthy Eating for Life to Prevent and Treat Cancer, ISBN 047143597X

Physicians Committee for Responsible Medicine, Healthy Eating for Life for Children, ISBN 0471436216

Physicians Committee for Responsible Medicine, Healthy Eating for Life for Women, ISBN 0471435961

Plant, Jane and Tidey, Jill, Understanding, Preventing and Overcoming Osteoporosis, ISBN 1852270772

Pritikin, Nathan, The Pritikin Program for Diet and Exercise, 0867530049

Rogers, Sandy, Fruit & Vegetables as Medicine, ISBN 0646388878

Schlosser, Eric, Fast Food Nation, ISBN 0713996021

Stafford, Julie, Juicing for Health, ISBN 0670906476

Stepaniak, Joanne (MS), Being Vegan, ISBN 1737303239

Taylor, Ross, Creating Health, Yourself, ISBN 0646308750

Virkler, Mark & Patti, Go Natural, ISBN 1560431385

Walker, Norman (DSc), Fresh Vegetable & Fruit Juices, ISBN 08901906704

Walker, Norman (DSc), Colon Health: The Key to Vibrant Life, ISBN 0890190690

Videos

Klaper, Michael (MD), A Diet For All Reasons - Dr Michael Klaper, Video. In this powerful one hour presentation, Dr. Michael Klaper demonstrates how the foods we eat can either support our health or contribute to disease. This video is by far the most powerful evidence to convince anyone that we should be eating only plant-based foods. Do you have friends or relatives you want to help go vegetarian, vegan or to just eat healthier? This video has influenced more people to stop or cut back on eating meat and dairy products than any other video we know of. Logical, scientific, easy to understand and convincing.

Web Sites

Cancer Project. To make cancer prevention a top priority of modern medicine. To uncover vital links between cancer and environmental factors, especially dietary links. To educate the public and provide individuals with tools shown to dramatically reduce cancer risk. www.cancerproject.org

Christian Vegetarian Association. To support and encourage Christian vegetarians around the world. To share with non-vegetarian Christians how a vegetarian diet can add meaning to one's faith, aid in one's spirituality, and enhance one's moral life. To show the world that the gospel of Jesus Christ is good news for both humans and animals by living a consistent Christian life of peace and non-violence toward all God's creatures. www.christianveg.com

Eat Veg. A good resource site, but maybe a little too commercial. Lots of terrific articles and information. www.eatveg.com

Modern Manna. Christian health education and gospel ministry. www.modernmanna.org

Veg Source. To offer the most up to date health and diet information possible, and to encourage the many good reasons for a plant-based diet. They do this by sponsoring leading authorities and organizations and promoting their critical message. www.vegsource.com

APPENDIX B
DEFINITIONS

Acid: A solution containing H+ ions and has a pH between 0 and 7.

Alkaline: A chemical compound that contains OH- ions or absorbs H+ ions when dissolved in water. **Alkalines** have a pH between 7 and 14.

Amino Acid: Form the basic building blocks of proteins. Amino acids are formed from aminos (NH_2) and carboxylic acids (NOOH).

Base: See Alkaline.

Calorie: See kilojoule. As a rough guide, there are 4 calories per kilojoule (exact number is 4.1868).

Carbohydrate: Group of organic compounds that includes sugar, starch and cellulose. Carbohydrates contain the main energy source in the diet of man and animals. They are produced by photosynthesis in plants and contain carbon, hydrogen and oxygen atoms.

Carcinogen: A chemical known to cause tumors and cancers.

Cellulose: A complex carbohydrate composed of glucose units and forms the cell walls of plants.

Cholesterol: A white, waxy lipid synthesized by the liver.

Cholesterol consists of high density lipoproteins (HDL) and low density lipoproteins (LDL).

Disaccharide: Carbohydrate compound of two monosaccharides.

DNA: Deoxyribonucleic acid. A nucleic acid that contains genetic information in a cell and is capable of self-reproduction. DNA forms the now-familiar double helix molecule.

Enzyme: Number of proteins functioning as catalysts for internal biochemical reactions.

Ester: Class of organic compound formed from organic acids and alcohol. Common fats and oils are mixtures of esters formed from glycerol and fatty acids.

Fat: General term for various organic compounds constituting esters and fatty acids.

Fat - Hydrogenated: These are unsaturated fats that have been made saturated with hydrogen by heat or other chemical means. Margarine is a prime example of a partially hydrogenated fat.

Fat - Monounsaturated: Like unsaturated fat, but one pair of carbon atoms in the chain share a double bond rather than a single bond.

Fat - Polyunsaturated: Like unsaturated fat, but two or more carbon atom pairs contain a double bond and contain fewer hydrogen atoms than they can hold.

Fat - Saturated: Every available carbon atom contains a hydrogen atom, that is, saturated with hydrogen. Solid at room temperature, like lard or butter. Derived from animal sources and associated with high levels of cholesterol.

Fat - Unsaturated: Contain fewer hydrogen atoms than they can hold, with double bonds between carbon atoms. Liquid at room temperature, like olive oil. Derived from plant sources and do not contain any cholesterol.

Fatty Acids: Any long-chain organic acids derived from fats.

Fiber: Course, indigestible plant matter consisting mainly of complex carbohydrates and polysaccharides, such as cellulose. Also known as 'roughage'.

Free Radical: Atom that has at least one unpaired electron and is therefore highly unstable and reactive.

Glyceride: An ester of glycerol and fatty acid.

Glycerol: A sweet, syrupy fluid obtained from fats and oils. Often used as a base for moisturizers.

Glycogen: Polysaccharide forming the main carbohydrate storage in the liver and muscle tissues. Readily converts to glucose for energy.

Hydrogenation: The addition of hydrogen to a compound, in particular solidification of unsaturated fats to saturated fats.

Insulin: A peptide hormone secreted by the pancreas to regulate the metabolism of carbohydrates, fats and sugars. Active in the transmission of glucose from the bloodstream to the cells of the body.

Kilojoule: Unit of heat energy under the international metric system of measurement. A kilojoule is 1000 joules, where a joule is the amount of energy expended when a 1 kg mass is accelerated at 1 m/s^2 for a distance of 1 meter.

Linoleic Acid: An essential fatty acid.

Lipid: Name given to organic fats, oils, waxes and triglycerides that are insoluble in water.

Lipoprotein: Conjugated organic proteins comprised of both proteins and lipids. Lipoproteins are the main carriers of lipids in the bloodstream.

Mineral: Elements of the periodic table such as calcium, potassium, sodium, iron, zinc, etc, that are essential to human growth and body functions.

Monosaccharide: A class of sugar that cannot be broken down into simpler forms.

Omega-3, Omega-6: Both are essential polyunsaturated fatty acids, since they must be obtained from food. While it is true that fish and fish oils provide copious amounts of these fatty acids, eating fish is not recommended due to the high protein, fat and cholesterol levels associated with their flesh. Plant sources rich in omega-3's and 6's are nuts (walnuts, brazil nuts, hazelnuts), sesame seeds, chick peas (and humus dip made from chick peas), and leafy green vegetables.

Peristalsis: Wavelike muscular contractions that moves material through the intestines.

pH: pH = $-\log_{10}$[H+], that is, minus log to the base 10 of the concentration of H+ ions in solution.

Photosynthesis: Process in green plants by which carbohydrates are converted from carbon dioxide and water using light energy. Oxygen is released as a by-product.

Polysaccharide: Class of carbohydrates such as starch and cellulose consisting mainly of chains of monosaccharides.

Protein: Chemical compounds comprised of carbon, hydrogen, oxygen, nitrogen and sulfur. Proteins are comprised of long chains of amino acids.

Radical: Group of elements or atoms that can pass through one compound to another but generally incapable of existing in a free state for very long.

RNA: Ribonucleic acid. RNA determines protein synthesis and transmission of genetic information.

Saccharide: Any compound of carbon, hydrogen and oxygen in which the hydrogen and oxygen atoms exist in a ratio of 2:1. This includes many sugars.

Starch: An abundant carbohydrate found in plants, particularly tubers such as potatoes.

Sugar: A general term for carbohydrate crystalline substances having a sweet taste. A general term for sugars such as glucose, fructose, galactose, maltose, sucrose lactose and saccharides.

Sugar - Fructose: Sugar occurring in fruits and honey.

Sugar - Galactose: Monosaccharide occurring in lactose and some pectins.

Sugar - Glucose: Monosaccharide occurring widely in plant cells. Principle sugar in the bloodstream and source of energy for the body.

Sugar - Lactose: Disaccharide found in dairy. Also known as 'milk sugar'.

Sugar - Sucrose: Dissaccharide of fructose and glucose found in plants.

Tissue: Aggregation of similar cells acting together to perform specific functions. Includes muscle, nerve, membranes and connective tissue.

Triglyceride: Fat-like substances that are carried through the bloodstream. Most of the body's fat is stored as triglycerides that can be used as energy. So called because triglyceride molecules consist of three fatty acids.

Vitamin: Various fat-soluble and water-soluble organic substances required in minute quantities for normal growth and body function.

APPENDIX C
VEGGIE QUOTATIONS

Christian Barnard (MD): I had bought two male chimps from a primate colony in Holland. They lived next to each other in separate cages for several months before I used one as a heart donor. When we put him to sleep in his cage in preparation for the operation, he chattered and cried incessantly. We attached no significance to this, but it must have made a great impression on his companion, for when we removed the body to the operating room, the other chimp wept bitterly and was inconsolable for days. The incident made a deep impression on me. I vowed never again to experiment with such sensitive creatures.

Neal Barnard (MD): The beef industry has contributed to more American deaths than all the wars of this century, all natural disasters, and all automobile accidents combined. If beef is your idea of 'real food for real people,' you'd better live real close to a real good hospital.

Drew Barrymore: The thing that has been weighing on my mind this week is that I wanted to go and save all the little live lobsters in restaurants and throw them back in the ocean. Imagine me being arrested for that.

Saint Basil: The steam of meat meals darkens the spirit. One can hardly have virtue if one enjoys meat meals and feasts. In the earthly paradise there was no wine, no one sacrificed animals, and no one ate meat.

Kim Bassinger: If you could see or feel the suffering you wouldn't think twice. Give back life. Don't eat meat.

Catherine Booth: The awful cruelty and terror to which tens of thousands of animals killed for human food are subjected in traveling long distances by ship and rail and road to the slaughter-houses of the world. God disapproves of all cruelty, whether to man or beast. The occupation of slaughtering animals is brutalizing to those who are required to do the work.... I believe this matter is well worthy of the serious consideration of Christian leaders.

William Booth: It is a great delusion to suppose that flesh-meat of any kind is essential to health. Considerably more than three parts of the work in the world is done by men who never taste anything but vegetable, farinaceous food, and that of the simplest kind. There are more strength-producing properties in wholemeal flour, peas, beans, lentils, oatmeal, roots, and other vegetables of the same class, than there are beef or mutton, poultry or fish, or animal food of any description whatever.

Kate Bush: People's general awareness is getting much better, even down to buying a pint of milk: the fact that the calves are actually killed so that the milk doesn't go to them but to us cannot really be right, and if you have seen a cow in a state of extreme distress because it cannot understand why its calf isn't by, it can make you think a lot.

T. Colin Campbell (MD): Usually, the first thing a country does in the course of economic development is to introduce a lot of livestock. Our data are showing that this is not a very smart move and the Chinese are listening. They are realizing that animal-based agriculture is not the way to go.... We are basically a vegetarian species and should be eating a wide variety of plant food and minimizing our intake of animal foods.... Once people start introducing animal products into their diet, that's when the mischief starts.

Rachel Carson: Until we have the courage to recognize cruelty for what it is - whether its victim is human or animal - we cannot expect things to be much better in this world... We cannot have peace among men whose hearts delight in killing any living creature. By every act that glorifies or even tolerates such moronic delight in killing we set back the progress of humanity.

William Castelli (MD): Vegetarians have the best diet. They have the lowest rates of coronary disease of any group in the country. Some people scoff at vegetarians, but they have a fraction of our heart attack rate and they have only 40 percent of our cancer rate. They outlive other men by about six years now.

William Castelli (MD): When you see the golden arches you are probably on your way to the pearly gates.

Peter Cheeke: Do we, as humans, having an ability to reason and to communicate abstract ideas verbally and in writing, and to form ethical and moral judgments using the accumulated knowledge of the ages, have the right to take the lives of other sentient organisms, particularly when we are not forced to do so by hunger or dietary need, but rather do so for the somewhat frivolous reason that we like the taste of meat? In essence, shouldn't we know better?

Saint Clement: It is far better to be happy than to have your bodies act as graveyards for animals. Accordingly, the apostle Matthew partook of seeds, nuts and vegetables, without flesh. *St Clement.*

James Cromwell: If any kid ever realized what was involved in factory farming they would never touch meat again. I was so moved by the intelligence, sense of fun and personalities of the animals I worked with on Babe that by the end of the film I was a vegetarian.

Doris Day: Killing an animal to make a coat is sin. It wasn't meant to be, and we have no right to do it. A woman gains status when she refuses to see anything killed to be put on her back. Then she's truly beautiful.

John Denver: Many things made me become a vegetarian, among them the higher food yield as a solution to world hunger.

Clint Eastwood: I take vitamins daily, but just the bare essentials not what you'd call supplements. I try to stick to a vegan diet heavy on fruit, vegetables, tofu, and other soy products.

Albert Einstein: Nothing will benefit human health and increase chances for survival of life on Earth as much as the evolution to a vegetarian diet. If a man aspires towards a righteous life, his first act of abstinence is from injury to animals.

Francis of Assisi: All things of creation are children of the Father and thus brothers of man, God wants us to help animals, if they need help. Every creature in distress has the same right to be protected. If you have men who will exclude any of God's creatures from the shelter of compassion and pity, you will have men who deal likewise with their fellow men. Not to hurt our humble brethren is our first duty to them, but to stop there is not enough. We have a higher mission - to be of service to them wherever they require it.

Benjamin Franklin: Flesh eating is unprovoked murder.

Richard Gere: People get offended by animal rights campaigns. It's ludicrous. It's not as bad as mass animal death in a factory.

Vincent van Gogh: Since visiting the abattoirs of southern France I have stopped eating meat.

Geoffrey Giuliano (played Ronald McDonald but quit in 1980): I brainwashed youngsters into doing wrong. I want to say sorry to children everywhere for selling out to concerns who make millions by murdering animals.

Werner Hartinger (MD): Vivisection is barbaric, useless, and a hindrance to scientific progress.

Thomas Jefferson: Until we stop harming all other living beings, we are still savages. I have lived temperately, eating little animal food, and not as an aliment, so much as a condiment for the vegetables which constitute my principle diet.

Saint Jerome: The eating of meat was unknown up to the big flood, but since the flood they have the strings and stinking juices of animal meat into our mouths, just as they threw in front of the grumbling sensual people in the desert. Jesus Christ, who appeared when the time had been fulfilled, has again joined the end with the beginning, so that it is no longer allowed for us to eat animal meat.

William Kellog: How can you eat anything with eyes?

Michael Klaper (MD): There is strong medical evidence that complete freedom from eating animal flesh or cow's milk products is a gateway to optimal nutritional health. All red meat contains saturated fat. There is no such thing as truly lean meat. Trimming away the edge ring of fat around a steak really does not lower the fat content significantly. People who have red meat (trimmed or untrimmed) as a regular feature of their diets suffer in far greater numbers from heart attacks and strokes.

The Dalai Lama: Killing animals for sport, for pleasure, for adventure, and for hides and furs is a phenomena which is at once disgusting and distressing. There is no justification in indulging is such acts of brutality.

C. S. Lewis: If we cut up beasts simply because they cannot prevent us and because we are backing our own side in the struggle for existence, it is only logical to cut up imbeciles, criminals, enemies, or capitalists for the same reasons.

Abraham Lincoln: I am in favor of animal rights as well as human rights. That is the way of a whole human being.

Howard Lyman: Most Americans don't have any idea how well the Department of Agriculture protects the grower at the expense of the consumer. When a chemical is banned from use, a farmer or livestock operator who has the chemical in stock has a choice: either to lose money by disposing of the product, or to use it and take the risk of getting caught breaking the law. How severe is that risk? Well, if you use a banned product in your cattle feed, you have to face the prospect that the government is going to inspect one out of every 250,000 carcasses. They will test this carcass not for all banned substances, but just for a small fraction of them. And even if they detect some residue of a banned substance, and even if they're able to trace the carcass to the ranch that produced it, the guilty rancher is likely at most to receive a stern letter with a strongly worded warning. I never met a rancher who suffered in any way from breaking any regulation meant to protect the safety of our meat. The whole procedure is, in short, a charade.

Paul McCartney: The medical argument for animal testing doesn't stand up. Even if it did, I don't think we should kill other species. We think we're so much better; I'm not sure we are. I tell people, We've beaten into submission every animal on the face of the Earth, so we are the clear winners of whatever battle is going on between the species. Couldn't we be generous? I really do think it's time to get nice. No need to keep beating up on them. I think we've got to show that we're kind.

Martina Navratilova: I haven't bought any leather articles for a very long time. My ideal is to be able to avoid all animal products, in food as well as clothing.

Dean Ornish (MD): I don't understand why asking people to eat a well-balanced vegetarian diet is considered drastic, while it is medically conservative to cut people open and put them on cholesterol-lowering drugs for the rest of their lives.

Gary Player: The closer you can live to being a vegetarian the better.

Plutach: Can you really ask what reason Pythagoras had for abstaining from flesh? For my part I rather wonder both by what accident and in what state of soul or mind the first man did so, touched his mouth to gore and brought his lips to the flesh of a dead creature, he who set forth tables of dead, stale bodies and ventured to call food and nourishment the parts that had little before bellowed and cried, moved and lived. How could his eyes endure the slaughter when throats were slit and hides flayed and limbs torn from limb? How could his nose endure the stench? How was it that the pollution did not turn away his taste, which made contact with the sores of others and sucked juices and serums from mortal wounds? It is certainly not lions and wolves that we eat out of self-defense; on the contrary, we ignore these and slaughter harmless, tame creatures without stings or teeth to harm us, creatures that, I swear, Nature appears to have produced for the sake of their beauty and grace. But nothing abashed us, not the flower-like like tinting of the flesh, not the persuasiveness of the harmonious voice, not the cleanliness of their habits or the unusual intelligence that may be found in the poor wretches. No, for the sake of a little flesh we deprive them of sun, of light, of the duration of life to which they are entitled by birth and being.

Natham Pritikin: Vegetarians always ask about getting enough protein. But I don't know any nutrition expert who can plan a diet of natural foods resulting in a protein deficiency, so long as you're not deficient in calories. You need only 5 or 6 percent of total calories in protein... and it is pratically impossible to get below 9 percent in ordinary diets.

Pythagoras: The earth affords a lavish supply of riches, of innocent foods, and offers you banquets that involve no bloodshed or slaughter. Only beasts satisfy their hunger with flesh, and not even all of those, because horses, cattle, and sheep live on grass.

William Roberts (MD): When we kill the animals to eat them, they end up killing us because their flesh, which contains cholesterol and saturated fat, was never intended for human beings.

Romain Rolland: To a man whose mind is free there is something even more intolerable in the sufferings of animals than in the sufferings of man. For with the latter it is at least admitted that suffering is evil and that the man who causes it is a criminal. But thousands of animals are uselessly butchered every day without a shadow of remorse. If any man were to refer to it, he would be thought ridiculous. And that is the unpardonable crime

George Bernard Shaw: Atrocities are not less atrocities when they occur in laboratories and are called medical research. Animals are my friends-and I don't eat my friends.

Jerry Seinfeld: Who was the first person to drink milk, and what were they thinking? Ooo boy, I can't wait 'til those calves get done so I can get me a shot of that.

Peter Singer: Those who, by their purchases, require animals to be killed have no right to be shielded from the slaughterhouse or any other aspect of the production of the meat they buy. If it is distasteful for humans to think about, what can it be like for the animals to experience it?

Steven Spielberg: Humans are the only hunters who kill when not hungry.

Robert Louis Stephenson: Nothing more strongly arouses our disgust than cannibalism, yet we make the same impression on Buddhists and vegetarians, for we feed on babies, though not our own.

Leo Tolstoy: A human can be healthy without killing animals for food. Therefore if he eats meat he participates in taking animal life merely for the sake of his appetite.

Mark Twain: I am not interested to know whether vivisection produces results that are profitable to the human race or doesn't...The pain which it inflicts upon unconsenting animals is the basis of my enmity toward it, and it is to me sufficient justification of the enmity without looking further.

Mary Tyler-Moore: As a civilized nation, we have an ethical obligation to prevent animal cruelty and to treat animals, including farm animals, as sentient beings. In doing so, we prevent intolerable suffering, and we elevate the human spirit.

Leonardo da Vince: One day the world will look upon research upon animals as it now looks upon research on human beings.

Richard Wagner: If experiments on animals were abandoned on grounds of compassion, mankind would have made a fundamental advance.

John Wesley: Thanks be to God! Since the time I gave up the use of flesh-meats and wine, I have been delivered from all physical ills.

Walter Willet (MD): If you step back and look at the data, the optimum amount of red meat you eat should be zero.

APPENDIX D
SCIENTIFIC STUDIES

T hese studies were obtained from the National Center for Biotechnology Information, established in 1988 as a national resource for molecular biological information. One of the functions of NCBI is to provide public databases, including medical publications. The NCBI website is www.ncbi.nlm.nih.gov.

Cancer Studies

Food, Nutrition, and the Prevention of Cancer: A Global Perspective

American Cancel Council Report, American Institute for Cancer Research (AICR) and the World Cancer Research Fund.

In addition to emphasizing increased consumption of vegetables, fruits, legumes, and grain-based foods, which have been shown to have a protective effect particularly for cancers of the gastrointestinal and respiratory tracts, the report highlights the importance of staying physically active and maintaining a healthy body weight. The American Cancer Society concurs with these recommendations with only minor exceptions. In the area of physical activity the Society recommends at least 30 minutes of moderate physical activity on most days of the week, while the global report calls for one hour of physical activity every day. Studies have shown that physical activity can help protect against some cancers, either by balancing caloric intake with energy expenditure or by other mechanisms. An imbalance of caloric intake and output can lead to overweight, obesity, and increased risk for cancers at several sites, including colorectal, prostate, endometrium, breast (among postmenopausal women) and kidney.

Galactose consumption and metabolism in relation to the risk of ovarian cancer.

Cramer DW, Harlow BL, Willett WC, Welch WR, Bell DA, Scully RE, Ng WG, Knapp RC. Brigham and Women's Hospital, Obstetrics and Gynecology Epidemiology Center, Boston, Massachusetts 02115.PMID: 2567871

In a case-control study, consumption of dairy foods by 235 white women with epithelial ovarian cancer and by 239 control women, and activity of red blood cell galactose-1-phosphate uridyl transferase (transferase) in a subset of 145 cases and 127 controls were determined. Yogurt was consumed at least monthly by 49% of cases and 36% of controls. The mean transferase activity of cases was significantly lower than that of controls. When a ratio of lactose consumption to transferase (L/T) was calculated, cases had a mean L/T of 1.17 compared with 0.98 for controls; there was a highly significant trend for increasing ovarian cancer risk with increasing L/T ratio. Lactose consumption may be a dietary risk factor and transferase a genetic risk factor for ovarian cancer.

Epidemiology of prostate cancer with special reference to the role of diet.

Hirayama T. PMID: 537622

A prospective epidemiologic study of prostate cancer was conducted in Japan. The 10-year follow-up study of 122,261 men aged 40 years and above, who constitute 94.5% of the census population of 29 Health Center Districts, revealed a significantly lower age-standardized death rate for prostate cancer in men who daily ate green and yellow vegetables. This association is consistently observed in each age-group, in each socioeconomic class, and in each prefecture. Selected epidemiologic phenomena, such as the upward trend of the prostate cancer death rate in Japan, intracountry variation of death rate, the significantly lower incidence rate in Japan compared with that of the United States, and elevated risk in Japanese migrants to Hawaii, appear to be explained by the variation in diet and change in amount of green and yellow vegetables ingested. The possible role of vitamin A is considered as a factor in preventing and inhibiting growth of prostate cancer. Most of the other factors studied appear noncontributory, except for marital status; a higher risk was observed in "ever married" men.

Dietary factors and the incidence of cancer of the stomach.

Risch HA, Jain M, Choi NW, Fodor JG, Pfeiffer CJ, Howe GR, Harrison LW, Craib KJ, Miller AB. PMID: 2998182.

A case-control study of diet and stomach cancer was conducted during 1979-1982 in Toronto, Winnipeg, and St. John's Canada. Two hundred forty-six histologically verified cancer cases were individually matched by age, sex, and area of residence to 246 randomly selected population controls. Daily nutrient consumption values were calculated from quantitative diet history questionnaire data through use of the US Department of Agriculture Food Composition Data Bank, which was extended and modified for Canadian items. For the analysis, continuous conditional logistic regression methods were used. It was found that consumption of dietary fiber was associated with decreased risk of gastric cancer; the odds ratio estimate of trend was 0.40/10 g average daily intake of fiber (i.e., 0.40(1.5)/15 g, etc.) (p less than 10(-8)). Also, average daily consumption of nitrite, chocolate, and carbohydrate was associated with increasing trends in risk, with odds ratio estimates, respectively, 2.6/mg (p less than 10(-4)), 1.8/10 g (p less than 10(-4)), and 1.5/100 g (p = 0.015). While citrus fruit intake appeared to be somewhat protective (odds ratio =

0.75/100 g daily average, p = 0.0056), vitamin C intake was less so, and vitamin E not at all. Thus, a number of dietary components seem to be implicated in the pathogenesis of stomach cancer.

Role of fat, animal protein, and dietary fiber in breast cancer etiology: a case-control study.

Lubin F, Wax Y, Modan B. PMID: 3018342

A case-control study of 818 breast cancer (BC) patients and 2 matched control groups, surgical controls (SCs) and neighborhood controls (NCs), was undertaken in Israel between 1975 and 1978. The interview schedule included a detailed dietary history based on the frequency of consumption of 250 food items, which were grouped according to their principal nutrient component. The average frequency of consumption of each food item in each nutrient group was computed. Medical, demographic, hormonal, and parity histories were also obtained. Risks associated with fat, animal protein, and fiber consumption were evaluated. Two types of analysis were performed [in 2 age groups (less than 50 yr and greater than or equal to 50 yr)], using the conditional logistic method: evaluating the risk attributable to nutrition only and controlling for nondietary confounding factors as well. When no adjustment for nondietary confounding factors was made, the risk increased with fat intake in both age groups [one-tailed P-value for linear trend = .08 and .07 in age less than 50 and .01 and .10 for the greater than or equal to 50 age category for the BC case (BCC)-SC and BCC-NC comparisons, respectively]. Increased fiber intake decreased the risk in the younger age group (one-tailed P-value for linear trend = .06 and .07 for the BCC-SC and BCC-NC comparisons, respectively), while in the 50-or-over age category the trend was inconsistent. The risk associated with animal protein was much less clear. For women in the highest quartiles of fat and animal protein intake and the lowest quartiles of fiber intake, risk was about twice as high as that for women in the lowest quartiles of fat and animal protein intake and in the highest quartile of fiber intake (one-tailed P-value for linear trend = .04 and .08 for age less than 50 and .08 and .09 for the age category greater than or equal to 50 BCC-SC and BCC-NC comparisons, respectively). When hormonal and demographic confounding factors were controlled for, this pattern persisted but it remained significant for 1 control only. Power increased when cases were analyzed against both controls simultaneously (one-tailed P-value for linear trend = .10 for age less than 50 and .02 for age greater than or equal to 50). <u>Thus a higher fat-animal protein and lower fiber diet is associated with increased cancer risk, but this relationship needs to be studied further.</u>

Physical activity and cancer etiology: associations and mechanisms.

McTiernan A, Ulrich C, Slate S, Potter J. Fred Hutchinson Cancer Research Center, Cancer Prevention Research Program, Seattle, WA 98104, USA. PMID: 9934715.

OBJECTIVES: This paper reviews the epidemiologic data of associations between physical activity and cancer risk, describes potential mechanisms for a physical activity cancer link, and proposes future directions for research. METHODS: We reviewed English-language published papers on physical activity and cancer through Medline searches for epidemiologic studies, and through references on individual reports. We reviewed general texts on effects of exercise on human biology and applied the concepts to the biology of cancer in humans to describe potential mechanisms for a physical activity-cancer association. RESULTS: <u>Considerable epidemiologic evidence has accrued linking increased physical activity with reduced occurrence of cancers of the breast and colon.</u> The association between physical activity and cancers of other sites is unclear. Potential mechanisms for the association between physical activity and reduced risk for breast and colon cancer are varied: they range from bias due to physical activity's strong correlations with other health factors (e.g., diet, smoking, alcohol use, use of medications) to the metabolic effects resulting from increased physical activity and fitness, such as reduced obesity, hormonal and reproductive effects, mechanical effects, and enhancement of the immune system. CONCLUSIONS: <u>The elucidation of biologic mechanisms for an association between physical activity and cancer may provide biological support for the association.</u> It will contribute information to determine the type, frequency, and duration of exercise needed to maximize protection. This information will be needed before large-scale community interventions are begun, in order to choose the correct interventions for the desired effect of reduced incidence of the most common cancers.

Diabetes Studies

Cow milk and insulin-dependent diabetes mellitus: is there a relationship?

Scott FW, Nutrition Research Division Food Directorate, Health & Welfare Canada, Ottawa Ontario. PMID: 2309656.

Various cow-milk preparations have, with some variation, been reported to be diabetogenic in two animal models of insulin-dependent diabetes mellitus (IDDM), the BioBreeding (BB) rat and the nonobese diabetic (NOD) mouse. However, the suggestion of an inverse relationship between breast-feeding and IDDM based on epidemiological studies, remains controversial. <u>There is a significant positive correlation between consumption of unfermented milk protein and incidence of IDDM in data from various countries. Conversely, a possible negative relationship is observed between breast-feeding at age 3 mo and IDDM risk. Diet may be an important permissive factor in the development of IDDM.</u>

A bovine albumin peptide as a possible trigger of insulin-dependent diabetes mellitus.

Karjalainen J, Martin JM, Knip M, Ilonen J, Robinson BH,

Savilahti E, Akerblom HK, Dosch HM.Hospital for Sick Children, Department of Pediatrics and Immunology, University of Toronto, ON, Canada.PMID: 1377788

BACKGROUND. <u>Cow's milk has been implicated as a possible trigger of the autoimmune response that destroys pancreatic beta cells in genetically susceptible hosts, thus causing diabetes mellitus.</u> Studies in animals have suggested that bovine serum albumin (BSA) is the milk protein responsible, and an albumin peptide containing 17 amino acids (ABBOS) may be the reactive epitope. Antibodies to this peptide react with p69, a beta-cell surface protein that may represent the target antigen for milk-induced beta-cell—specific immunity. METHODS. We used immunoassays and Western blot analysis to analyze anti-BSA antibodies in the serum of 142 children with insulin-dependent diabetes mellitus, 79 healthy children, and 300 adult blood donors. Anti-ABBOS antibodies were measured in 44 diabetic patients at the time of diagnosis, three to four months later, and one to two years later. RESULTS. All the diabetic patients had elevated serum concentrations of IgG anti-BSA antibodies (but not of antibodies to other milk proteins), the bulk of which were specific for ABBOS. The mean (+/- SE) concentration was 8.5 +/- 0.2 kilofluorescence units (kfU) per microliter, as compared with 1.3 +/- 0.1 kfU per microliter in the healthy children. IgA antibodies were elevated as well, but not IgM antibodies. The antibody concentrations declined after diagnosis, reaching normal levels in most patients within one to two years. The initial decline involved anti-ABBOS—specific antibodies almost exclusively. Much lower serum concentrations of anti-BSA antibodies were found in all 379 control subjects, but only 2.5 percent of them had small amounts of ABBOS-specific IgG. CONCLUSIONS. <u>Patients with insulin-dependent diabetes mellitus have immunity to cow's-milk albumin,</u> with antibodies to an albumin peptide that are capable of reacting with a beta-cell—specific surface protein. Such antibodies could participate in the development of islet dysfunction.

Postprandial serum glucose, insulin, and lipoprotein

responses to high- and low-fiber diets.

Anderson JW, O'Neal DS, Riddell-Mason S, Floore TL, Dillon DW, Oeltgen PR. Metabolic Research Group, Veterans Affairs Medical Center, Lexington, KY 40511, USA. PMID: 7616842

The effects of high-fiber (HF) and low-fiber (LF) meals on postprandial serum glucose, insulin, lipid, lipoprotein, and apolipoprotein concentrations of 10 hypercholesterolemic men were examined using a random-order, cross over design. HF and LF meals provided 15% of energy as protein, 40% as carbohydrate, and 45% as fat, 200 mg cholesterol/1,000 kcal, and 25 g fiber/1,000 kcal for HF or 3 g fiber/1,000 kcal for LF. Responses over a 15-hour period after multiple meals (MM) and over a 10-hour period after a single meal (SM) were compared. HF meals were associated with a significant reduction in postprandial serum glucose (P < .0005 after SM) and insulin (P < .0005 after SM). Serum free fatty acid (FFA) levels decreased significantly after MM and SM, but differences between HF and LF meals were insignificant. Although serum triglyceride responses did not differ significantly (ANOVA) between HF and LF meals, values were higher at 2 and 3 hours after a HF SM than after a LF SM and at 16 hours after HF MM than after LF MM. Although serum cholesterol values did not differ significantly (ANOVA) between HF and LF meals, values were higher after a HF SM than after a LF SM. Other subtle differences in responses of high-density lipoprotein (HDL) cholesterol, HDL2, and HDL3 concentrations were noted. These studies indicate that large increases in dietary fiber intake are accompanied by small changes in postprandial serum lipoprotein concentrations.

Dietary fiber, glycemic load, and risk of NIDDM in men.

Salmeron J, Ascherio A, Rimm EB, Colditz GA, Spiegelman D, Jenkins DJ, Stampfer MJ, Wing AL, Willett WC. Department of Nutrition, Harvard School of Public Health, Boston, Massachusetts 02115, USA. PMID: 9096978

OBJECTIVE: Intake of carbohydrates that provide a large glycemic response has been hypothesized to increase the risk of NIDDM, whereas dietary fiber is suspected to reduce incidence. These hypotheses have not been evaluated prospectively. RESEARCH DESIGN AND METHODS: We examined the relationship between diet and risk of NIDDM in a cohort of 42,759 men without NIDDM or cardiovascular disease, who were 40-75 years of age in 1986. Diet was assessed at baseline by a validated semiquantitative food frequency questionnaire. During 6-years of follow-up, 523 incident cases of NIDDM were documented. RESULTS: The dietary glycemic index (an indicator of carbohydrate's ability to raise blood glucose levels) was positively associated with risk of NIDDM after adjustment for age, BMI, smoking, physical activity, family history of diabetes, alcohol consumption, cereal fiber, and total energy intake. Comparing the highest and lowest quintiles, the relative risk (RR) of NIDDM was 1.37 (95% CI, 1.02-1.83, P trend = 0.03). Cereal fiber was inversely associated with risk of NIDDM (RR = 0.70; 95% CI, 0.51-0.96, P trend = 0.007; for > 8.1 g/day vs. < 3.2 g/day). The combination of a high glycemic load and a low cereal fiber intake further increased the risk of NIDDM (RR = 2.17, 95% CI, 1.04-4.54) when compared with a low glycemic load and high cereal fiber intake. CONCLUSIONS: These findings support the hypothesis that diets with a high glycemic load and a low cereal fiber content increase risk of NIDDM in men. Further, they suggest that grains should be consumed in a minimally refined form to reduce the incidence of NIDDM.

Does a vegetarian diet reduce the occurrence of diabetes?

Snowdon DA, Phillips RL. PMID: 3985239

We propose the hypothesis that a vegetarian diet reduces the risk of developing diabetes. Findings that have generated this hypothesis are from a population of 25,698 adult White Seventh-day Adventists identified in 1960. During 21 years of follow-up, the risk of diabetes as an underlying cause of death in Adventists was approximately one-half the risk for all US Whites. <u>Within the male Adventist population, vegetarians had a substantially lower risk than non-vegetarians of diabetes as an underlying or contributing cause of death. Within both the male and female Adventist populations, the prevalence of self-reported diabetes also was lower in vegetarians than in non-vegetarians.</u> The associations observed between diabetes and meat consumption were apparently not due to confounding by over- or under-weight, other selected dietary factors, or physical activity. All of the associations between meat consumption and diabetes were stronger in males than in females.

Toward improved management of NIDDM: A randomized, controlled, pilot intervention using a lowfat, vegetarian diet.

Nicholson AS, Sklar M, Barnard ND, Gore S, Sullivan R, Browning S. Physicians Committee for Responsible Medicine, Georgetown University Medical Center, Washington, DC, USA. PMID: 10446033

OBJECTIVE: To investigate whether glycemic and lipid control in patients with non-insulin-dependent diabetes (NIDDM) can be significantly improved using a low-fat, vegetarian (vegan) diet in the absence of recommendations regarding exercise or other lifestyle changes. METHODS: Eleven subjects with NIDDM recruited from the Georgetown University Medical Center or the local community were randomly assigned to a low-fat vegan diet (seven subjects) or a conventional low-fat diet (four subjects). Two additional subjects assigned to the control group failed to complete the study. The diets were not designed to be isocaloric. Fasting serum glucose, body weight, medication use, and blood pressure were assessed at baseline and biweekly thereafter for 12 weeks. Serum lipids, glycosylated hemoglobin, urinary albumin, and dietary macronutrients were assessed at baseline and 12 weeks. RESULTS: Although the sample was intentionally small in accordance with the pilot study design, the 28% mean reduction in fasting serum glucose of the experimental group, from 10.7 to 7.75 mmol/L (195 to 141 mg/dl), was significantly greater than the 12% decrease, from 9.86 to 8.64 mmol/L (179 to 157 mg/dl), for the control group (P < 0.05). The mean weight loss was 7.2 kg in the experimental group, compared to 3. 8 kg for the control group (P < 0.005). <u>Of six experimental group subjects on oral hypoglycemic agents, medication use was discontinued in one and reduced in three. Insulin was reduced in both experimental group patients on insulin. No patient in the control group reduced medication use.</u> Differences between the diet groups in the reductions of serum cholesterol and 24-h microalbuminuria did not reach statistical significance; however, high-density lipoprotein concentration fell more sharply (0.20 mmol/L) in the experimental group than in the control group (0.02 mmol/L) (P < 0.05). CONCLUSION: <u>The use of a low-fat, vegetarian diet in patients with NIDDM was associated with significant reductions in fasting serum glucose concentration and body weight in the absence of recommendations for exercise.</u> A larger study is needed for confirmation.

Heart Disease Studies

Can lifestyle changes reverse coronary heart disease?

Ornish D, Brown SE, Scherwitz LW, Billings JH, Armstrong WT, Ports TA, McLanahan SM, Kirkeeide RL, Brand RJ, Gould KL, Pacific Presbyterian Medical Center, Sausalito, California. PMID: 1973470.

In a prospective, randomised, controlled trial to determine whether comprehensive lifestyle changes affect coronary atherosclerosis after 1 year, 28 patients were assigned to an experimental group <u>(low-fat vegetarian diet, stopping smoking, stress management training, and moderate exercise)</u> and 20 to a usual-care control group. 195 coronary artery lesions were analysed by quantitative coronary angiography. The average percentage diameter stenosis regressed from 40.0 (SD 16.9)% to 37.8

(16.5)% in the experimental group yet progressed from 42.7 (15.5)% to 46.1 (18.5)% in the control group. When only lesions greater than 50% stenosed were analysed, the average percentage diameter stenosis regressed from 61.1 (8.8)% to 55.8 (11.0)% in the experimental group and progressed from 61.7 (9.5)% to 64.4 (16.3)% in the control group. <u>Overall, 82% of experimental-group patients had an average change towards regression. Comprehensive lifestyle changes may be able to bring about regression of even severe coronary atherosclerosis after only 1 year, without use of lipid-lowering drugs.</u>

Epidemiology of coronary heart disease: the Framingham study.

Castelli WP. PMID: 6702862

Coronary heart disease continues to be the number one cause of death in most Northern European, North American and other industrialized Caucasian societies. By the age of 60, every fifth man and one in 17 women have some form of this disease. One in 15 men and women will eventually have a stroke. Other cardiovascular diseases related to atherosclerosis are also important. Epidemiologic (prospective) studies enable one to predict most of the potential victims of cardiovascular disease, years before they become ill. <u>An increase in total to high-density lipoprotein cholesterol ratio, hypertension, cigarette smoking, excess weight, elevated blood sugar levels, lack of exercise, stress, electrocardiographic abnormalities, and other factors are associated with the development of these diseases.</u> Intervention trials have generally shown that lowering "risk factors" reduces the subsequent rate of coronary heart disease, stroke, and other cardiovascular disease. Most highly susceptible subjects have problems with several risk factors. Management of one should not interfere with management of another if optimal health is sought.

Lowering Blood Cholesterol To Prevent Heart Disease

National Institutes of Health, Consensus Development Conference

Statement, December 10-12, 1984

Elevated blood cholesterol level is a major cause of coronary artery disease. It has been established beyond a reasonable doubt that lowering definitely elevated blood cholesterol levels (specifically blood levels of low-density lipoprotein cholesterol) will reduce the risk of heart attacks due to coronary heart disease. This has been demonstrated most conclusively in men with elevated blood cholesterol levels, but much evidence justifies the conclusion that similar protection will be afforded in women with elevated levels. After careful review of genetic, experimental, epidemiologic, and clinical trial evidence, we recommend treatment of individuals with blood cholesterol levels above the 75th percentile (upper 25 percent of values). Further, we are persuaded that the blood cholesterol level of most Americans is undesirably high, in large part because of our high dietary intake of calories, saturated fat, and cholesterol. In countries with diets lower in these constituents, blood cholesterol levels are lower, and coronary heart disease is less common. There is no doubt that appropriate changes in our diet will reduce blood cholesterol levels. Epidemiologic data and over a dozen clinical trials allow us to predict with reasonable assurance that such a measure will afford significant protection against coronary heart disease.

Osteoporosis Studies

Milk, dietary calcium, and bone fractures in women: a 12-year prospective study.

Feskanich D, Willett WC, Stampfer MJ, Colditz GA. Channing Laboratory, Boston, Mass. 02115, USA. PMID: 9224182.

OBJECTIVES: This study examined whether higher intakes of milk and other calcium-rich foods during adult years can reduce the risk of osteoporotic fractures. METHODS: This was a 12-year prospective study among 77761 women, aged 34 through 59 years in 1980, who had never used calcium supplements. Dietary intake was assessed with a food-frequency questionnaire in 1980, 1984, and 1986. Fractures of the proximal femur (n = 133) and distal radius (n = 1046) from low or moderate trauma were self-reported on biennial questionnaires. RESULTS: We found no evidence that higher intakes of milk or calcium from food sources reduce fracture incidence. Women who drank two or more glasses of milk per day had relative risks of 1.45 for hip fracture (95% confidence interval [CI] = 0.87, 2.43) and 1.05 for forearm fracture (95% CI = 0.88, 1.25) when compared with women consuming one glass or less per week. Likewise, higher intakes of total dietary calcium or calcium from dairy foods were not associated with decreased risk of hip or forearm fracture. CONCLUSIONS: These data do not support the hypothesis that higher consumption of milk or other food sources of calcium by adult women protects against hip or forearm fractures.

Dietary influences on bone mass and bone metabolism: further evidence of a positive link between fruit and vegetable consumption and bone health?

New SA, Robins SP, Campbell MK, Martin JC, Garton MJ, Bolton-Smith C, Grubb DA, Lee SJ, Reid DM - Center for Nutrition and Food Safety, School of Biological Sciences, University of Surrey, Guildford, United Kingdom. PMID: 10617959.

BACKGROUND: The role of nutritional influences on bone health remains largely undefined because most studies have focused attention on calcium intake. OBJECTIVE: We reported previously that intakes of nutrients found in abundance in fruit and vegetables are positively associated with bone health. We examined this finding further by considering axial and peripheral bone mass and markers of bone metabolism. DESIGN: This was a cross-sectional study of 62 healthy women aged 45-55 y. Bone mineral density (BMD) was measured by dual-energy X-ray absorptiometry at the lumbar spine and femoral neck and by peripheral quantitative computed tomography at the ultradistal radial total, trabecular, and cortical sites. Bone resorption was calculated by measuring urinary excretion of pyridinoline and deoxypyridinoline and bone formation by measuring serum osteocalcin. Nutrient intakes were assessed by using a validated food-frequency questionnaire; other lifestyle factors were assessed by additional questions. RESULTS: After present energy intake was controlled for, higher intakes of magnesium, potassium, and alcohol were associated with higher total bone mass by Pearson correlation ($P < 0.05$ to $P < 0.005$). <u>Femoral neck BMD was higher in women who had consumed high amounts of fruit in their childhood than in women who had consumed medium or low amounts</u> ($P < 0.01$). In a regression analysis with age, weight, height, menstrual status, and dietary intake entered into the model, magnesium intake accounted for 12.3% of the variation in pyridinoline excretion and 12% of the variation in deoxypyridinoline excretion. Alcohol and potassium intakes accounted for 18.1% of the variation in total forearm bone mass. CONCLUSION: <u>The BMD results confirm our previous work (but at peripheral bone mass sites), and our findings associating bone resorption with dietary factors provide further evidence of a positive link between fruit and vegetable consumption and bone health.</u>

Case-control study of risk factors for hip fractures in the elderly.

Cumming RG, Klineberg RJ, Department of Public Health, University of Sydney, NSW, Australia. PMID: 8154473

The objective of this population-based case-control study was to identify risk factors for hip fracture among elderly women and men, particularly factors during young and middle adult life. The study base comprised people aged 65 years and over living in a defined region in Sydney, Australia, during 1990-1991. Cases were recruited from 12 hospitals, and controls were selected using an area probability sampling method, with additional sampling from nursing homes. There were 416 subjects (209 cases and 207 controls); proxy respondents were needed for 27 percent of the subjects. Smoking, underweight in old age, overweight at age 20 years, and weight loss were associated with an increased risk of hip fracture. <u>Consumption of dairy products, particularly at age 20 years, was associated with an increased risk of hip fracture in old age.</u> Multivariate-adjusted odds ratios for quintiles of dairy product consumption at age 20 years were 1.0 (lowest quintile), 0.8, 1.8, 3.4, 2.9 (highest quintile). Caffeine and alcohol intake were not associated with hip fracture risk. Some of the results of this study were unanticipated and may be due to chance or bias. If confirmed by other studies, these results would challenge some current approaches to hip fracture prevention.

Potassium, magnesium, and fruit and vegetable intakes are associated with greater bone mineral density in elderly men and women.

Tucker KL, Hannan MT, Chen H, Cupples LA, Wilson PW, Kiel DP, Jean Mayer US Department of Agriculture Human Nutrition Research Center on Aging at Tufts University, Boston, MA 02111, USA, PMID: 10197575

BACKGROUND: Osteoporosis and related fractures will be growing public health problems as the population ages. It is therefore of great importance to identify modifiable risk factors. OBJECTIVE: We investigated associations between dietary components contributing to an alkaline environment (dietary potassium, magnesium, and fruit and vegetables) and bone mineral density (BMD) in elderly subjects. DESIGN: Dietary intake measures were associated with both cross-sectional (baseline) and 4-y longitudinal change in BMD among surviving members of the original cohort of the Framingham Heart Study. Dietary and supplement intakes were assessed by food-frequency questionnaire, and BMD was measured at 3 hip sites and 1 forearm site. RESULTS: Greater potassium intake was significantly associated with greater BMD at all 4 sites for men and at 3 sites for women ($P < 0.05$). Magnesium intake was associated with greater BMD at one hip site for both men and women and in the forearm for men. Fruit and vegetable intake was associated with BMD at 3 sites for men and 2 for women. Greater intakes of potassium and magnesium were also each associated with less decline in BMD at 2 hip sites, and greater fruit and vegetable intake was associated with less decline at 1 hip site, in men. There were no significant associations between baseline diet and subsequent bone loss in women. CONCLUSION: These results support the hypothesis that alkaline-producing dietary components, specifically, potassium, magnesium, and fruit and vegetables, contribute to maintenance of BMD.

A high ratio of dietary animal to vegetable protein increases the rate of bone loss and the risk of fracture in post-menopausal women. Study of Osteoporotic Fractures Research Group.

Sellmeyer DE, Stone KL, Sebastian A, Cummings SR. Division of Endocrinology, the General Clinical Research Center, and the Department of Epidemiology and Biostatistics, University of California, San Francisco, USA. PMID: 11124760

BACKGROUND: Different sources of dietary protein may have different effects on bone metabolism. Animal foods provide predominantly acid precursors, whereas protein in vegetable foods is accompanied by base precursors not found in animal foods. Imbalance between dietary acid and base precursors leads to a chronic net dietary acid load that may have adverse consequences on bone. OBJECTIVE: We wanted to test the hypothesis that a high dietary ratio of animal to vegetable foods, quantified by protein content, increases bone loss and the risk of fracture. DESIGN: This was a prospective cohort study with a mean (+/-SD) of 7.0+/-1.5 y of follow-up of 1035 community-dwelling white women aged >65 y. Protein intake was measured by using a food-frequency questionnaire and bone mineral density was measured by dual-energy X-ray absorptiometry. RESULTS: Bone mineral density was not significantly associated with the ratio of animal to vegetable protein intake. Women with a high ratio had a higher rate of bone loss at the femoral neck than did those with a low ratio (P = 0.02) and a greater risk of hip fracture (relative risk = 3.7, P = 0.04). These associations were unaffected by adjustment for age, weight, estrogen use, tobacco use, exercise, total calcium intake, and total protein intake. CONCLUSIONS: Elderly women with a high dietary ratio of animal to vegetable protein intake have more rapid femoral neck bone loss and a greater risk of hip fracture than do those with a low ratio. This suggests that an increase in vegetable protein intake and a decrease in animal protein intake may decrease bone loss and the risk of hip fracture. This possibility should be confirmed in other prospective studies and tested in a randomized trial.

A High Ratio of Dietary Animal to Vegetable Protein Increases the Rate of Bone Loss and the Risk of Fracture in Postmenopausal Women

Sellmeyer DE, Stone KL, Sebastian A, et al. American Journal of Clinical Nutrition. 2001;73:118-122

The hypothesis that a high dietary ratio of animal protein to vegetable protein increases bone loss and risk of fracture was studied in a prospective cohort of 1035 women who participated in the Study of Osteoporotic Fractures (SOF). White community-dwelling women were recruited for the study and were aged > 65 years. Recent dietary history (over the preceding 12 months) was assessed using a "validated" food frequency questionnaire. Intakes of protein were calculated from this questionnaire. BMD was measured using DXA at the total hip and subregions. Two BMD measurements were taken with an average of 3.6 years (SD 0.4 years) between each assessment. The rate of bone loss was calculated as the percentage difference between 2 BMD measurements in a subset of the participants (n = 742). Hip fractures were assessed prospectively for 7 years (SD 1.5 years), and fracture data were available for all the 1035 women for whom the dietary data were collected. Fractures were confirmed with radiographs and a review of the radiologist reports. Results were intriguing. Women with a higher ratio of animal to vegetable protein intake had a higher rate of bone loss at the femoral neck than did those with a low ratio, as well as a greater risk of hip fracture (relative risk = 3.7). These findings remained significant after adjustment for important confounding factors, including age, weight, estrogen use, tobacco use, physical activity, and total Ca and protein intake. These findings provide further support for a link between vegetable-based proteins and indices of bone health and suggest that a decrease in animal protein and an increase in vegetable protein may decrease bone loss and risk of hip fracture.

APPENDIX E
AUSTRALIAN DATA

This appendix gives equivalent statistics and data found in the text for Australia. The relevant page to which the data relates to is also referenced.

Chapter 1 — Marvelous Are His Works

Page 26: The following table shows the number of deaths by disease in Australia in the year 2002...[1]

Disease	No. Deaths	Percent
Malignant neoplasms (cancer)	37,458	28.2%
Ischaemic heart disease	25,884	19.5%
Cerebrovascular disease (stroke)	12,459	9.4%
Chronic lower respiratory diseases	6,246	4.6%
Accidents	4,877	3.7%
Diabetes mellitus	3,296	2.5%
Influenza and pneumonia	3,063	2.3%
Arterial diseases	2,634	2.0%

Chapter 2 — The Genesis Diet

Page 35: In Australia, the total health expenditure in 2002-03, from all sources, was estimated at AUD$72.2 billion, 9.5% of Gross Domestic Product (GDP) or AUD$3,652 per person. In terms of health expenditure as a proportion of GDP and expenditure per person, Australia has spent at an increasing rate compared to the OECD average in the past decade.[2]

Page 35: According to the Australian Bureau of Statistics, the population of Australians over 65 years of age will be 4.2 million in 2021 and between 6.4 and 6.8 million by 2051. As a proportion of population, this will represent and increase from 12% in 1999 to 18-19% in 2021 and 25-28% in 2051.[3]

Page 36: On the basis of prevailing cancer incidence rates, it is expected that one in three men and one in four women in Australia will be directly affected by cancer before the age of 75.[4]

Page 39: In Australia, 68% of men and 52% of women are overweight or obese, representing about 7 million people, or 35% of the population. By 2020, it is estimated that 75% of the Australian population will be overweight or obese.[5]

Page 78: In Australia, some 1.2 million people have diabetes. It is the 6th highest cause of death, and is estimated to cost AUD$3 billion annually.[6]

1. **Australian Bureau of Statistics**, 3303.0 Causes of Death, www.abs.gov.au

2. **Australian Institute of Health and Welfare**, www.aihw.gov.au

3. **Australian Demographic Statistics**, Looking Into the Future,

Australian Population Projections, March 2000, www.abs.gov.au

4. **Australian Institute of Health and Welfare**, Cancer in Australia 1996 Report, www.aihw.gov.au

5. **Victorian Government, Better Health Channel**, Obesity. www.betterhealthchannel.com.au

6. **Diabetes Australia**, Diabetes Facts, www.dav.org.au

APPENDIX F
REFERENCES

Chapter 1 — Marvelous Are His Works

1. **Reader's Digest** - Family Health Guide, page 24. ISBN 090948662X

2. **Genetech**, DNA Structure, www.gene.com

3. **University of California**, Berkeley, Museum of Paleontology, Ernst Haeckel, www.ucmp.berkeley.edu

4. Estimates for the number of cells in the body vary, but is most certainly in the order of trillions

5. **National Human Genome Research Institute**, www. genome.gov

6. **Albuminous**: A class of simple, water-soluble proteins that can be coagulated by heat, such as egg-whites

7. **Minnesota State University**, The Skeletal System, www.mnsu.edu

8. Ibid

9. **Education Foundation**, Muscular System, library.think quest.org

10. **The Franklin Institute Online**, Oxygen Delivery System, sln.fi.ed

11. **A Look Inside the Human Body**, The Respiratory System, www4.tpgi.com.au

12. **The Franklin Institute Online**, The Circle of Blood, sln.fi.edu

13. **Biology Online**, Leucocytes, www.biology-online.org

14. **The Medem Network**, The Lymphatic System, www.medem. com

15. **University of Oxford**, Nuffield Department of Anaesthetics, The Automonic Nervous System by Dr S Blackwell, Adden-brooke's Hospital, Cambidge, www.nda.ox.ac.uk

16. **MemoryZine**, How Does the Brain Work? www.memory zine.com

17. **National Digestive Diseases Information Clearing House**, Your Digestive System and How it Works, digestive.niddk.nih.gov

18. **Moorehead State University**, Human Anatomy, Lecture Notes 21, people.morehead-st.edu

19. **Health Square**, The Reproductive System, www.health-square.com

20. **Guinness Book of Records**, Edition 1999, page 102

21. **Medical News Today**, www.medicalnewstoday.com

22. **Centers for Disease Control and Prevention**, National Vital Statistics Reports, Vol 53, No 17, Deaths and Percentage of Total Deaths for the 10 Leading Causes of Death, 2002, www.cdc.gov

23. **Dr. Alexander Leaf**, National Geographic, January, 1973

24. **Dr Allen Banik**, Hunza Land

25. **Venderbilt Faculty & Staff Wellness Program**, Longevity

May Have Spiritual Link, vanderbiltowc.wellsource.com

26. **University of Texas**, Population Research Center, Religious Involvement and US Adult Mortality, Hummer RA, Rogers RG, Nam CB, Ellison CG, PMID: 10332617, www.ncbi.nlm.nih.gov

Chapter 2 — The Genesis Diet

1. **Eric Schlosser**, Fast Food Nation, page 113, ISBN 0713996021

2. **Seventh Day Adventist**, International Journal of Faith, Thought and Action, Healthy Choices and Living Options, dialogue.adventist.org

3. **Dr Sidney Katz**, University of British Columbia

4. **Columbia Encyclopedia**, Volume 18, page 5355

5. **MedTerms Online Medical Dictionary**, Penicillin History, www.medterms.com

6. **National Network for Immunization Information**, Vaccines and Diseases They Prevent, www.immunization.org

7. **OECD**, Health Spending in Most OECD Countries Rises, With the US Far Outstripping All Others, www.oecd.org

8. **Center for Medicare and Medicaid Services**, www.cms. hhs.gov

9. **Second World Assembly on Ageing**, Madrid, Spain, April, 2002, www.un.org

10. **U.S. Census Bureau**, National Population Projections, www.census.gov

11. **American Cancer Society**, Cancer Burden is Expected to Rise with an Ageing Population, www.cancer.org

12. **Dr John McDougall**, MD, The McDougall Program for a Healthy Heart, page 206

13. Ibid, page 210-211

14. Ibid, page 207

15. **Jenny Bryan and John Clare**, Organ Farm, page 21, ISBN 184222249X

16. **Oak Ridge National Laboratory**, What are Genetically Modified Foods? www.ornl.gov

17. Ibid

18. **Science Controversies Online Partnerships in Education (SCOPE)**, Who Benefits from the Products of GM Foods, scope.educ.washington.edu

19. **American Obesity Association**, AOA Fact Sheets, www.obesity.org

20. **National Institute of Health**, hin.nhlbi.nih.gov/portion/

21. **Better Health Channel**, www.betterhealth.vic.gov.au

22. **The Age**, Obesity Epidemic May Reduce Life Span, March 19, 2005. Article quotes paper published in the New England Journal of Medicine by Professor Jay Olshansky

23. **Dr Neal Barnard, MD**, Food for Life, page 88, ISBN 0517882019

24. **The Diet Channel**, Analysis of the Atkins Diet, www.thedietchannel.com

25. **An Introduction to the Atkins Diet**, weightloss.about.com

26. **PCRM**, Atkins Diet Alert, www.atkinsdietalert.org

27. **PCRM**, Judge Again Rules in Favor of Man Suing Atkins Empire, www.pcrm.org/news/health050105.html

28. **University of Florida**, Journalism and Communications, Food Pyramid History, www.iml.jou.ufl.edu

29. Ibid

30. Ibid

31. **Harvard School of Public Health**, What Should You Really Eat? www.hsph.harvard.edu

32. **Health News Website**, Building a Better Food Pyramid, www.healthnewswebsite.com

33. **United States Department of Agriculture**, My Pyramid, www.mypyramid.gov

34. **PCRM**, www.pcrm.org

35. **Dr Neal Barnard, MD**, Food for Life, page 143

36. **CNN**, Legumes: An Alternative to Meat, June 17, 2003, www.cnn.com

37. **Henry Ford Museum**, Soybean Experimental Laboratory, www.hfmgv.org

38. **Omega Engineering Inc**, Introduction to pH, www.omega.com

39. **Dr Joel Robbins**, www.learnhealth.org

40. **Ross Taylor**, Creating Health Yourself, page 42, ISBN 064630870

41. **Dr Neal Barnard, MD**, Food for Life, page 3, ISBN 0517882019

42. Ibid, page 73

43. **BBC News**, How Cats' Eyes Helped Change The World, July 22, 2002, news.bbc.co.uk

44. **Linus Pauling Institute**, Micronutrient Information Center, lpi.oregonstate.edu

45. **MedicineNet**, Age Related Macular Degeneration, www.medterms.com

46. **Why Nutrients Called Flavonoids are Good For You**, www.nutritionreporter.com

47. **Dr Ray Sahalien**, MD, www.raysahelian.com

48. **Harvard School of Public Health**, www.hsph.harvard.edu

49. **Vegetarian Resource Group**, Calcium in the Vegan Diet, www.vrg.org

50. **Christiaan Eijkman Biography**, www. nobelprize.org

51. **Rosemary Stanton**, Fat & Fiber Counter, ISBN 1863501193. A look up of unprocessed meats, chicken, fish and eggs shows a fiber content of zero.

52. **Canadian Diabetes Association**, The Benefits of Eating Fiber, www.diabetes.ca

53. **Dr Norman Walker**, Colon Health, The Key to a Vibrant Life, page 3

54. **Columbia University Department of Surgery**, Colorectal Cancer, www.columbiasurgery.org

55. **American Heart Association**, Cholesterol, www.american-heart.org

56. **Dr Neal Barnard, MD**, Turn off the Fat Genes, page 59, ISBN 073291096X

57. **Allan Borushek**, Pocket Calorie and Fat Counter, page 5, ISSN 13259970

58. **Dr John McDougall, MD**, The McDougall Program for a Healthy Heart, page 38, ISBN 0525938680

59. **PCRM**, Cholesterol and Heart Disease, www.pcrm.org

60. **Whole Health MD**, Amino Acids, www.wholehealthmd.com

61. **Bombay Hospital Journal**, Food Values of a Vegetarian Diet, www.bhj.org

62. **John Robbins**, Diet for A New America, page 173, ISBN 0915811812

63. Ibid, page 177

64. **Dairy Australia**, www.dairyaustralia.com.au

65. **Professor Jane Plant and Gill Tidey**, Understanding, Preventing and Overcoming Osteoporosis, page viii

66. **FAOSTAT** (Food and Agricultural Organization of the United Nations), an online database containing food and agricultural statistics.

67. **University of Washington**, Osteoporosis and Bone Physiology, www. courses.washington.edu

68. **National Institute of Diabetes and Digestive and Kidney Diseases**, Lactose Intolerance, digestive.niddk.nih.gov

69. **Swiss Lab Pty Ltd**, Fat Content Determination During Milk Standardization, www.developtechnology.com

70. **Abelow BJ, Holford TR, Insogna KL.**, Cross-cultural Association Between Dietary Animal Protein and Hip Fracture: a hypothesis, Yale University School of Medicine, PMID: 1739864.

71. **John Robbins**, Diet for A New America, page 192, ISBN 0915811812

72. **Dr Dean Ornish, MD**, Dr Dean Ornish's Program for Reversing Heart Disease, page 258

73. **Dr John McDougall, MD**, The McDougall Program for a Healthy Heart, page 78

74. **Framingham Heart Study**, www.framingham.com

75. Ibid

76. **Vegetarian Starter Kit**, by www.goveg.com

77. **Cancer Research UK**, What is Cancer? www.cancerre-searchuk.org

78. **American Cancer Society**, Children Surviving Cancer Need Follow Up, www.cancer.org

79. **Dr Don Colbert, MD**, Toxic Relief, page 7

80. **Dr Mitchell Gaynor, MD**, Dr Gaynor's Cancer Prevention Program, page 9, ISBN 1575663821

81. **US National Cancer Institute**, Understanding Cancer Series: The Immune System, www.cancer.gov

82. **Harvard School of Public Health**, Fruit, Vegetables and Cancer, www.hsph.harvard.edu

83. **The Cancer Project, Diet and Nutrition Facts**, Foods for Cancer Prevention, www.cancerproject.org

84. **PCRM**, Healthy Eating for Life to Prevent and Treat Cancer, page 12, ISBN 047143597X

85. **The American Cancer Society**, www.cancer.org

86. **PCRM**, Healthy Eating for Life to Prevent and Treat Diabetes, page 4, ISBN 0471435988

87. **American Diabetes Association**, National Diabetes Fact Sheet, www.diabetes.org

88. **Centers for Disease Control and Prevention**, National Vital Statistics Reports, Vol 53 No 17, Deaths and Percentage of Total Deaths for the 10 Leading Causes of Death, 2002, www.cdc.gov

89. **Diabetic Helper Organization**, www.diabetichelper.com

90. **PCRM**, Healthy Eating for Life to Prevent and Treat Diabetes, page 19, ISBN 0471435988

91. **American Diabetic Association**, Using the Diabetes Food Pyramid, www.diabetes.org

92. **PCRM**, Healthy Eating for Life to Prevent and Treat Diabetes, page 54, ISBN 0471435988

93. **David Jackson, B. Pharm, PhD, and Rayner Soothill, MSc**, Is the Medicine Making You Ill? page 13, ISBN 0207157960

94. **Dr Jay Cohen, MD**, Medication Sense, www.medication-sense.com

95. **Direct-to-Consumer Advertising & Prescription Drug Promotion**, marketreports.com

96. **Dr Randall Stafford, MD**, Stanford News Service, Pharmaceutical Companies Spent Millions Marketing Questionable Hormone Therapies, www.news-service.stanford.edu

97. **Dr Jay S. Cohen, M.D.**, Over Dose, The Case Against the Drug Companies, page 14

98. **Medline Plus**, National Library of Medicine, Drug Abuse and Dependence, www.nlm.nih.gov

99. **Medicinal Food News**, A Banana a Day Keeps the Doctor Away, www.medicinalfoodnews.com

100. **USA Weekend**, Bravo for Broccoli, February 3, 1995, www.usaweekend.com

101. **Dr Benjamin Lau, MD**, Garlic for Health, page 40, ISBN 0941524329

102. **Dr Don Colbert, MD**, Toxic Relief, page 150, ISBN 0884197603

103. **Dr Neal Barnard, MD**, Foods that Fight Pain, page 3, ISBN 0553812378

104. **American Macular Degeneration Foundation**, Improved Nutrition May Reduce the Risk of Macular Degeneration, www.macular.org/nutrition

105. **Experimental Biology and Medicine**, Tomatoes, Lycopene, and Prostate Cancer: Progress and Promise, www.ebmonline.org

Chapter 3 — Going Vegetarian

1. **American Dietetic Association**, Position Paper on Vegetarian Diets, 1997, www.eatright.org

2. **International Vegetarian Union**, History of Vegetarianism, www.ivu.org

3. famousveggie.com

4. **International Vegetarian Union**, History of Vegetarianism, www.ivu.org

5. **The Washington Times**, Analysis: Is Meat Packing a 'Jungle', washingtontimes.com

6. **McSpotlight**, Interview with Geoffrey Guiliano, www.mcspotlight.org

7. **Dr Alan Attwood, MD**, Dr Attwood's Low-Fat Prescription for Kids, ISBN 0140236449

8. **Dr Benjamin Spock, MD**, Article found on Physician's Committee for Responsible Medicine website, www.pcrm.org

9. **Dr Linda Palmer, DC**, Dynamic Chiropractic, May 1999

10. **Wright State University School of Medicine**, Lifespan Health Research Center, Department of Community Health, Kettering, OH 45420 USA. Early Menarche and the Development of Cardiovascular Disease (CVD) Risk Factors in 11. Adolescent Girls: the Fels Longitudinal Study. Remsberg KE, Demerath EW, Schubert CM, Chumlea C, Sun SS, Siervogel RM.. PMID: 15728207

11. **Dr Norman Walker**, Fresh Vegetable and Fruit Juices, page 3, ISBN 08901906704

12. **The Comparative Anatomy of Eating**, by Dr Milton R. Mills, MD, www.vegsourse.com

13. **Vegetarian and Vegan Foundation, UK**, www.vegetarian.org.uk

14. **British Broadcasting Corporation**, Monarchs & Leaders, King Henry VIII, www.bbc.co.uk

15. **Margarine and Spreads Association**, UK, www.margarine. org.uk

16. **Salt Institute**, www.saltinstitute.org

17. **Paul C. Bragg, ND, PhD**, The Miracle of Fasting. ISBN 0877900361

18. Ibid, page 15

19. **Salt Institute**, www.saltinstitute.org

20. **Eric Shlosser**, Fast Food Nation, ISBN 0713996021

21. **McDonald's Corporation**, The McDonald's History, www.mcdonalds.com

22. **Kentucky Fried Chicken**, Colonel Harland Sanders, www.kfc.com

23. **Kentucky Fried Chicken**, Original Recipe Is Still a Secret, www.kfc.com

24. **Center for Science In The Public Interest**, Fast Food Follow Up, www.cspinet.org

25. **CBS News**, Eat Less — Live Longer, August 1, 2002, www.cbsnews.com

26. **Parramatta City Council**, NSW, Litter Facts, www.parracity. nsw.gov.au

27. **Logan City Council**, QLD, Litter, www.logan.qld.gov.au

28. **The Age**, March 28, 2005, page 15. Article by Dr Rob Moodie, Chief Executive Officer of VicHealth, Australia

29. **McSpotlight**, McDonald's Censorship Strategy, www.mcspot-light.org

30. **New South Wales Parliament**, Legislative Council Hansard, Food Act 1989, Disallowance of Food Amendment (MSG)

Regulation 2002, www.parliament.nsw.gov.au

31. **Food Standards Australia New Zealand**, Food Additives, www.foodstandards.gov.au

32. **World Health Organization (WHO)**, Chemical Risks in Food, www.who.int

33. **Food Additives 'Cause Tantrums'**, BBC News, 25 October, 2002

34. **World Natural Health Organization**, Congressional Record, Aspartame, www.wnho.net

Chapter 4 — Other Important Factors

1. **Paul C. Bragg**, Water, The Shocking Truth, page 2, ISBN 0877900639

2. **Australian Natural Resource** Atlas, Water Use, audit.ea.gov. au/ANRA

3. **Harvard Medical School**, Increasing Risk From Waterborne Disease, www.med.harvard.edu

4. **Voice of America News Report**, Reporting of WHO Report, www.voanews.com

5. **Fluoridation**: A Horror Story: home1.gte.net/res0k62m/fluoride.htm

6. **Fluoride Action Group**, The Fog Disaster in the Meuse Valley, 1930: A Fluorine Intoxication, www.fluoridealert.org/meuse.htm

7. **Saskatchewan New Green Alliance**, Fluoride's Hidden History, www.nga.sk.ca/fluoride.html

8. **Fluoridation Status of Some Countries**, www.fluoridation. com/c-country.htm

9. **Paul C. Bragg**, Water — The Shocking Truth, page 153, ISBN 0877900639

10. **John Archer**, On the Water Front, page 28, ISBN 0646043188

11. Ibid, page 28

12. Ibid, page 30

13. **Paul C. Bragg**, Water, The Shocking Truth, page 7, ISBN 0877900639

14. **Bond University**, Faculty of Humanities and Social Sciences, Water Regulation and Drinking, www.hss.bond.edu.au

15. **Dr F. Batmanghelidj, MD**, Your Body's Many Cries for Water, page 7

16. **Dr Allen Banik, MD**, The Choice is Clear, page 15

17. **Dr Norman Walker**, Fresh Vegetable and Fruit Juices, page 7,ISBN 08901906704

Chapter 5 — Livestock Revolution

1. **Sustainable Agri-Food Production & Consumption**, Livestock Farms, www.agrifood-forum.net

2. **National Council for Science and the Environment**, Population and Sustainable Food Production, Propects for Food Security, www.cnie.org

3. **Vegetarian Network**, So Why Are You Still Eating Meat? (quoting Worldwatch Institute figures), www.vnv.org.au

4. **National Wild Turkey Federation**, Wild Turkey Facts, www.nwtf.org

5. **Time Magazine**, It's Not Too Early to Talk Turkey, September 8, 2003, www.time.com

6. **Humane Research Council** (AR Media), FarmStats Resource Page, www.armedia.org/farmstats.htm

7. **CBS News**, Peru Pushes Guinea Pigs as Food, October 19, 2004, www.cbsnews.com

8. **Free Farm Animals**, The Welfare of Hens in Battery Cages, www.freefarmanimals.org

9. **United Poultry Concerns**, Debeaking, www.upc-online.org

10. **Herbert Reed**, poultry producer, www.sentientbeings.org

11. **Poultry Science Organization**, Biochemical Analyses of Muscles from Poultry Bred for Rapid Growth, Department of Animal Sciences, Ohio State University, poultryscience.org

12. **Dr Michael Gregor, MD**, Latest in Human Nutrition, February, 2004, www.drgreger.org

13. **Pet Finder**, Back to the Future, www.petfinder.org

14. **Advocates for Animals**, The Facts About Broiler Chickens, www.advocatesforanimals.org.uk

15. **World Animal Foundation**, Factory Farming Fact Sheet, worldanimalfoundation.homestead.com

16. **A. B. Webster**, Department of Poultry Science, University of Georgia, Welfare Implications of Avian Osteoporosis, www.thep-oultrysite.com

17. **Justice Bell**, McDonalds vs Helen Steel and Dave Morris

18. **Eric Schlosser**, Fast Food Nation, page 140

19. **Richard Allison**, Department of Poultry Science, University of Georgia, Enriched Broilers, www.thepoultrysite.com

20. **The Observer**, Revealed, Horror at Tesco Pig Farm, October 19, 2003, observer.guardian.co.uk

21. **J. Messersmith**, Hog Farmer, www.sentientbeings.org

22. **Food Animals Concern Trust**, Factory Farming — The Odor is Just the Tip of the Iceberg, www.fact.cc

23. **J. Byrnes**, Hog Farm Management, 1976, www.sentientbe-ings.org

24. **The Veal Farm**, Pennsylvania Beef Council, Industry Information, www.vealfarm.com

25. **The Humane Society of the United States**, Veal Fact Sheet, www.hsus.org/farm_animals/

26. **Eazi-Breed CIDR Cattle Insert**, www.cidr.com

27. **Food Animals Concern Trust**, What is Happening to Dairy Cows, www.fact.cc/dairy_cows.htm

28. **Journal of Dairy Science**, Effects of Frequent Milking in Early Lactation on Milk Yield and Udder Health, www.dairy-science.org

29. **Food Animals Concern Trust**, What is Happening to Dairy Cows, www.fact.cc/dairy_cows.htm

30. **Food and Drug Administration (FDA)**, Commonly Asked Questions About BSE in Products Regulated by FDA's Center for Food Safety and Applied Nutrition (CFSAN), www.cfsan.fda.gov

31. **Howard Lyman**, About Howard, www.madcowboy.com

32. **Howard Lyman**, on the Oprah Winfrey Show, April, 1996

33. **CNN News**, Oprah Accused of Whipping up Anti-Beef 'Lynch Mob', January 21, 1998, www.cnn.com

34. **Find Law Resources** (Legal Resource on the Internet), Paul F. Engler, Cactus Feeders Inc. vs Oprah Winfrey, Harpo Productions and Howard Lyman, King World Productions, www.findlaw.com

35. **The Media Institute**, Libel Laws/Punitive Damages/Tort Actions, www.mediainstitute.org

36. **Washington Post**, Ex-Cattleman's Warning Was No Bum Steer, www.washingtonpost.com

37. **Human Rights Watch**, Blood, Sweat and Fear: Workers' Rights in US Meat and Poultry Plants, www.hrw.org

38. **Human Rights Watch**, Abuses Against Workers Taint U.S. Meat and Poultry, www.hrw.org

39. **Australian Trade Commission**, www.austrade.gov.au

40. **Australian Government**, Department of Agriculture, Fisheries and Wildlife, www.affa.gov.au

41. **Anglican Society for Welfare of Animals**, The Story of the Cormo Express, www.aswa.org.uk

42. **Royal Society for Prevention to Cruelty to Animals**, www.rspca.org.au

43. **John Howard, Prime Minister of Australia**, interview on radio 5DN, August 2003

44. **Australian Government, Department of Agriculture**, Fisheries and Forestry, www.affa.gov.au

45. Ibid

46. **Ethical Consumer**, Animal Testing Laboratories, www.ethicalconsumer.org

47. **The Body Shop** UK, Against Animal Testing — What's Happening in the UK, www.uk.thebodyshop.com

48. **EU Business**, EU Finally Set for Ban On Animal Testing in Cosmetics, www.eubusiness.com

49. **PCRM**, Position Paper on Animal Research, www.pcrm.org

50. **Vegan Society**, Feeding The World, www.vegansociety.com

51. **Food and Agricultural Organization of the United Nations**, Deforestation Continues at a High Rate in Tropical Areas, FAO Calls Upon Countries to Fight Forest Crime and Corruption, www.fao.org

52. **Canadian International Development Agency**, Forestry Advisers Network, Deforestation: Tropical Rainforests in Decline, www.rcfa-cfan.org

53. **Reuters**, April 1, 2004

54. **Dennis Avery**, Director of the Center of Global Food Issues, www.cgfi.org

55. **World Rainforest Movement**, What is the Underlying Cause of Deforestation, www.wrm.org.uy

56. **Physical Geography Net**, Introduction to the Atmosphere: The Greenhouse Effect. www.physicalgeography.net

57. **University of Wisconsin**, Deforestation in the Tropical Rainforests, www.uwsp.edu

58. **Michigan State University**, Center for Global Change & Earth Observations, Rain Forest Report Card, www.bsrsi.msu.edu

59. **John Robbins**, Diet for a New America, page 375, ISBN 0915811812

60. **International Vegetarian Association**, Animal Farming and the Environment, www.ivu.org

61. **Sierra Club**, America's oldest environmental organization, www.sierraclub.org

62. **Global Policy Forum**, Water — the Looming Source of World Conflict, March 20, 2001, www.globalpolicy.org

63. **Natural Resources Defense Council**, Cesspools of Shame: How Factory Farm Lagoons and Sprayfields Threaten Environmental and Public Health. www.nrdc.org

64. **Natural Resources Defense Council**, Report Documents Waste Lagoons' Threats to Environment, Public Health (Press Release), July 24, 2001, www.nrdc.org

65. **CNN**, Utility Knew of E. Coli Contamination But Did Nothing, archives.cnn.com

66. **Environment Protection Agency**, Animal Waste Management, Drinking Water Impacts, www.epa.gov

67. **Pittsburg Post-Gazzette**, October 16, 2003

68. **National Ocean Service**, Gulf of Mexico Hypoxia Assessment, www.nos.noaa.gov

69. **Environmental Defense**, Farm Bill Conservative Update-December 23, 2002, www.environmentaldefense.org

70. **Eric Schlosser**, Fast Food Nation, page 149

71. **The Scientific Alliance**, Research Race to Combat Wind, www.scientific-alliance.org

72. **Los Angeles Times**, July 13, 2003

73. **BBC News**, New Zealand Flatulence Tax Outrages Farmers, news.bbc.co.uk

74. **New Zealand Herald**, Livestock Burp Tax Sticks In Throat, June 20, 2003, www.nzherald.co.nz

75. **Sherwood Rowland**, University of California atmospheric chemist and Nobel Prize laureate, www.climateark.org

76. **Sustainable Table**, The Issues: Environment, www.sustainabletable.org/issues/environment

77. **MIT**, American Chemical Society Division of Chemical Toxicology, William Lijinsky, web.mit.edu

78. **Tasmanian Fishing Industry Council**, Dr Marcus Scammell, Environmental Problems — Georges Bay, Tasmania, www.tfic.com.au/scammell_report_07.04.htm

79. Ibid

Conclusion

1. **Dr Henry M. Morris**, The Genesis Record, page 78

INDEX

CPSIA information can be obtained
at www.ICGtesting.com
Printed in the USA
BVHW032029301020
592258BV00018B/49